D1590058

CHINESE *QIGONG* THERAPY

Compiled by
Zhang Mingwu
Sun Xingyuan

Translated by
Yang Entang
Yao Xiuqing

SHANDONG SCIENCE AND
TECHNOLOGY PRESS

JINAN, CHINA 1985

First Edition 1985

Published by THE SHANDONG SCIENCE AND
TECHNOLOGY PRESS

Binguan Xilu, Jinan, China

Printed by THE WEIFANG XINHUA PRINTING
HOUSE

99 Gongnong Road, Weifang, China

Distributed by CHINA INTERNATIONAL BOOK
TRADING CORPORATION

(GUOJI SHUDIAN)

P.O. Box 399, Beijing, China

Printed in the People's Republic of China

Acknowledgments

The translators wish to express their gratitude for the various kinds of help and advice they received from Mr. Shi Wencai, Mr. Sheng Wen, Mr. Han Gaoan, Dr. James J. Kohn and Mr. Slessor Scot.

Editor's Note

Qigong, one of the legacies in the treasure-house of Chinese medicine, has a history of three thousand years. It is an effective means of medical treatment as well as health protection with distinctive national features. It plays an active role in preventing and treating diseases, protecting and strengthening health, resisting premature senility and prolonging life. Particularly, it has unique effects in treating chronic and difficult diseases. That is why in ancient times Qigong was called "the method to eliminate diseases and prolong life". Self-controlled Qigong therapy is a method to control the body's function through Qigong practice and keep it under a stabilized appropriate state which is most favourable to overcoming the body's diseases. Qigong practice depends greatly on the practitioner's subjective initiative. It lays stress on: viewing the various parts of the human body as a whole, emphasizing the inner factors, taking both motion and quiescence into consideration, making the diagnosis and giving treatment on the basis of an overall analysis of the illness and of the patient's condition. It also emphasizes: organically combining mental daoyin, postural daoyin and breathing daoyin, proceeding from the easy to the difficult and from the exterior to the interior, progressing step by step in an orderly way and practising assiduously and

2

perseveringly so as to achieve the goal of training and fostering *Qi*, promoting the flow of internal *Qi*, maintaining a balance between *yin* and *yang*, dredging the channels and collaterals, regulating *Qi* and blood, treating diseases and protecting health, strengthening the body and prolonging life.

Now, *Qigong* is being accepted by more and more people. In order to help more people to master and apply the self-controlled *Qigong* therapy, Mr. Zhang Mingwu, adviser of All-China *Qigong* Research Association, vice-chairman of Eeijing *Qigong* Research Association, and others have written this "Self-Controlled *Qigong* Therapy" at our request.

This book introduces to the readers the writer's rich experience in *Qigong* practice by explaining to them the theory of self-controlled *Qigong* practice, the five basic *Qigong* patterns, the cancer-treating *Qigong* pattern, the hypertension-treating *Qigong* pattern, the massaging *Qigong* pattern, and some specific deviation-rectifying methods. To help the readers "suit the remedy to the case", some prescriptions for and case studies of some common diseases are arranged at the end of the book. Most of the cases reflect the writer's own experience in *Qigong* practice.

This book has substantial content. It is also easy to understand, to master and to apply. To read this book and practise *Qigong*, a healthy person can prolong his life and a weak person can eliminate his disease and strengthen his health. So it is a good teacher for the broad masses of people in terms of strengthening the body

We are grateful to Comrades Wu Qincheng, Yang Zongming, Zhu Baoshan, Zhu Yumei, Zheng Tingpan, Jiang Wenshu, Zhang Jingtian, Ye Peitong, Wang Tianbi, An Yunji, Zheng Qilin and Liu Zhijun for all the help they offered during the writing of this book.

1 9 8 5

Contents

1

7

Book I

THE PRINCIPLES
OF *QIGONG*

Chapter 1
Introduction

I. What is *Qigong*

Qigong is an art (a skill) of strengthening health practised typically in China. It plays an active role in preventing and treating diseases, protecting and strengthening health, resisting premature senility (decrepitude) and prolonging life. That is why *Qigong* was called the method "to eliminate diseases and prolong life" in ancient times.

Qi and *Gong* may be described separately as follows:

1. What is *Qi*

One always associates '*Qi*' with air. *Qi* includes "air" in its definition, but *Qi* must embody other meanings as well in the term *Qigong*.

According to results of tests performed by some scientists, the *Qi* released by a person who is skilled in the art of *Qigong* contains 'infrared radiation', 'static electricity', 'particle stream' and so on. According to the functions of *Qi* inside the human body, the *Qi* in *Qigong* is considered as a kind of message together with its carrier. And moreover, it is believed that the carrier is a kind of matter. So the *Qi* in *Qigong* does not only mean the inhaling of oxygen and exhaling of carbon dioxide, it also means a kind of matter that possesses a richer and more complicated message

3

and energy.

'Qi' is usually called 'internal Qi' or named as 'true Qi' by Qigong practitioners, to be differentiated from the air breathed in and out. Traditional Chinese medical theory holds that the 'true Qi' of the human body is the motive force of its vital activities. Therefore, the building up of Qi in terms of Qigong refers to the building up of true Qi.

True Qi can be classified into "Qi of the former heaven" (i.e., prenatal Qi) and "Qi of the latter heaven" (i.e., postnatal Qi). Prenatal Qi can be further classified into two forms—essential Qi (vital energy) and primordial Qi. Essential Qi refers to the bit of essential and vital energy that a human being obtains from the parents at the earliest stage of life, during the formation of the fetus. Primordial Qi denotes the fundamental matter and motive force that both maintain the physiological functions of the body's tissues and organs. During the development of fetus primordial Qi is already formed. It is stored in the kidney and is closely related with *the gate of life*. Postnatal Qi can also be classified into two kinds, i.e., heavenly Qi and earthly Qi. Heavenly Qi refers to the Qi we inhale and exhale. Earthly Qi means the Qi of water and grains. It is called earthly Qi because grains grow out of the earth. Actually it includes all the essential and fine Qis absorbed from various nutritious foods through the digestive system by our solid and hollow bodily organs to maintain vital activities. Only when filled with both heavenly Qi and earthly Qi, can the

4

human body carry on its vital activities.

While the prenatal Qi is the foundation, the motive force and is therefore indispensable, the postnatal Qi is the source of material for the vital activities of the body and is also indispensable. The relationship between the two kinds of Qi is: the prenatal Qi is the motive force of life and the postnatal Qi is the material on which life relies for its maintenance. A man's life and all his activities are motivated by the prenatal Qi and are supplemented by postnatal Qi. The two act on each other and rely upon each other, forming the true Qi for the body's vital activities.

2. What is *Gong*

Through *Qigong* exercise true Qi is made to function normally and exuberantly inside the human body—this is the meaning of *Gong*, usually called *Gongfu* in the term *Qigong*. The word *Gongfu* has broad implications. It may mean the time and quality of *Qigong* exercise, it may also mean the learning of methodology and attainment of skill in doing *Qigong* exercise. In short, it is a method to build up Qi.

A person's perseverance in doing *Qigong* exercise reflects his will power and determination. Neither doing it by fits and starts nor doing it without perseverance can produce good results. So the most important thing in doing *Qigong* exercise is perseverance.

The quality of doing *Qigong* exercise directly affects the results. The aim of doing *Qigong* exercise is to build up Qi, or, in other words, 'to foster the true Qi'. To have

5

sufficient true *Qi* means to be in excellent health. The building up of true *Qi* involves three modes of action (1) to breathe essential and vital *Qi*, (2) to maintain a quiescent mental state and (3) to keep the body organs in harmony ("Familiar Conversation" from *the Huang Di's Nei Jing*). These three modes of action are aimed at tempering the 'focus of thought', 'the breath' and 'the configuration' which are known as the three essential factors of *Qigong*.

3. The Technique of *Qigong* Exercise

The methods of *Qigong* exercise vary among different sects and schools. In China they are roughly classified into five schools—the Taoist School, the Buddhist School, the Confucian School, the Medical School and the Boxing School.

The method of the Taoist School considers strengthening 'both the body and the mind' as its dominant aim. The method is called 'to cultivate both life and nature', that is, to lay equal stress on practising *Qigong* and on contemplating nature.

The method of the Buddhist School 'lays emphasis on tempering the mind', i.e., giving no thought to the body.

The method of the Confucian School emphasizes 'regulating the mind'. 'sincerity' and 'cultivating' the moral character and urges the practitioner to reach the state of 'rest, calm and quiet'.

For the Medical School the main purpose in doing *Qigong* exercise is to treat diseases. But this school is also concerned with the promotion of health and prolongation of life.

The Boxing School gives emphasis on building up the

individual's strength against moral assaults and on attacking the enemy for self-protection. Although it also has the function of prolonging life in health protection, it differs greatly from the above-mentioned schools in preserving health.

Different as they are, the various methods of doing *Qigong* exercise can not go beyond the three broad kinds— the quiescent *Qigong*, the dynamic *Qigong* and the dynamic-quiescent *Qigong*. All of them involve three aspects of training—training the mind, training respiration and training the figure.

The training of the mental conditions involves the mental *daoyin* (guiding and inducing). It is required that the thoughts be concentrated on one object so as to put the cerebral cortex in a special inhibitory state. This is called 'the internal keeping of the mental state'.

The training of breathing refers to breathing *daoyin* (guiding and inducing). Breathing exercise includes exhaling, inhaling, breathing out deeply, blowing, aspirating and holding the breath.

The training of the figure means *daoyin* (guiding and inducing exercises) by various body positions. The postures are roughly divided into six kinds: walking, standing, sitting, lying, kneeling, and massaging.

No matter which method is to be followed, so long as the individual practises it consistently and follows its rules, he will certainly succeed in *Gong* in terms of *Gongfu*.

Ⅱ. **How Can *Qigong* Treat Diseases?**

1. Qi Flowing Along the Channels and Collaterals

The human body has a special system that connects the superficies with the interior, and the upper with the lower portions of the body and joins all the solid and hollow organs. Channels and collaterals are neither blood vessels nor nerves. The term channel (*jing*) has the meaning of "route". The channels are also called conduits of energy. They form the trunk lines. The term collateral (*luo*) has the meaning of network. The collaterals are branches of the channels. Channels and collaterals criss-cross the whole body and make the body into an organic unit by joining its various parts.

There are twelve regular channels—The Twelve Channels, leading to the solid and hollow organs. Their nature is expressed by the terms *yin* and *yang*. Those joining the solid organs and going along the interior laterals of the body are called *yin* channels. Those joining the hollow organs and going along the exterior laterals of the body are called *yang* channels. According to the nature of the viscera and the routes they follow, they are further classified as follows: three *yin* channels of the hand, three *yang* channels of thehand, three *yin* channels of the foot and three *yang* channels of the foot (see Table 1).

Table 1 The Twelve Channels

yin or yang / name of channel / hand or foot	Yin Channels Solid organs hold hollow organs (going along the interior laterals)	Yang Channels Hollow organs hold Solid organs (going along the exterior laterals)		body parts to pass through
hand	The Lung Channel of Hand-*Taiyin*	The Large Intestine Channel of Hand-*Yangming*	upper limbs	anterior line
hand	The Pericardium Channel of Hand-*Jueyin*	The Triple-Warmer Channel of Hand-*Shaoyang*	upper limbs	midline
hand	The Heart Channel of Hand-*Shaoyin*	The Small Intestine Channel of Hand-*Taiyang*	upper limbs	posterior line
foot	The Spleen Channel of Foot-*Taiyin*	The Stomach Channel of Foot-*Yangming*	lower limbs	anterior line→ midline
foot	The Liver Channel of Foot-*Jueyin*	The Gall Bladder Channel of Foot-*Shaoyang*	lower limbs	midline→ anterior line
foot	The Kidney Channel of Foot-*Shaoyin*	The Urinary Bladder Channel of Foot-*Taiyang*	lower limbs	posterior line

The flowing and joining rules of the twelve channels are as follows:

Three *yin* channels of hand extends from the chest and through the hand to join three *yang* channels of hand.

Three *yang* channels of hand extends from hand and through head to join three *yang* channels of foot.

Three *yang* channels of foot extends from head and through foot to join three *yin* channels of foot.

Three *yin* channels of foot extends from foot and through chest to join three *yin* channels of hand.

They are illustrated in the following sketch.

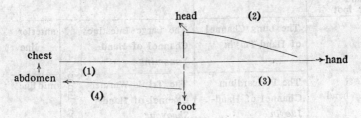

The Twelve Channels related to the solid and hollow organs

Yin channels are connected to solid organs and *yang* channels to hollow organs. When running through the viscera, the solid organs support the hollow organs in the case of *yin* channels and the hollow organs support the solid organs in the case of *yang* channels, thus forming six pairs of relationships unifying the superficies and interior.

The Twelve Channels cover the superficies and interior of the human body. Their flowing routes circulate through the body and are closely connected with each other (see Figures 1—12). They start from The Lung Channels of Hand-*Taiyin*, pass in turn to The Liver Channel of Foot-*Jueyin* and then to The Lung Channel of Hand-*Taiyin*. The two ends meet like a ring to complete the system.

For the relationship between the superficies and interior of the twelve channels and their flowing sequence, see

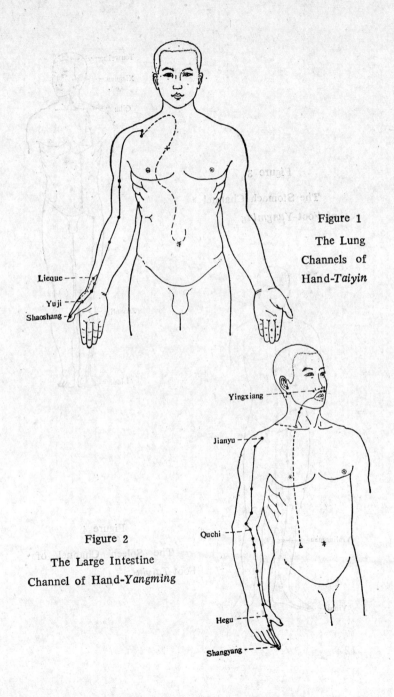

Figure 1

The Lung

Channels of

Hand-*Taiyin*

Lieque

Yuji

Shaoshang

Yingxiang

Jianyu

Quchi

Hegu

Shangyang

Figure 2

The Large Intestine

Channel of Hand-*Yangming*

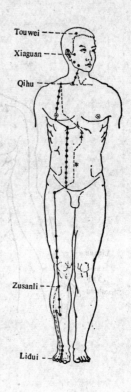

Touwei

Xiaguan

Qihu

Zusanli

Lidui

Figure 3

The Stomach Channel

of Foot-*Yangming*

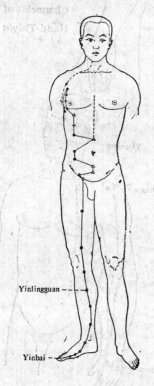

Yinlingguan

Yinbai

Figure 4

The Spleen Channel of

Foot-*Taiyin*

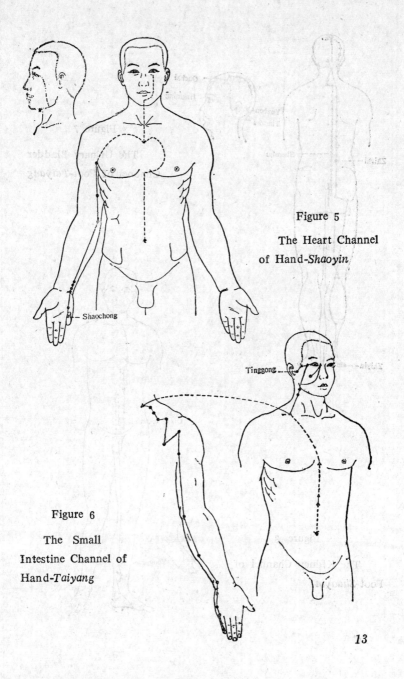

Figure 5

The Heart Channel
of Hand-*Shaoyin*

Shaochong

Tinggong

Figure 6

The Small
Intestine Channel of
Hand-*Taiyang*

13

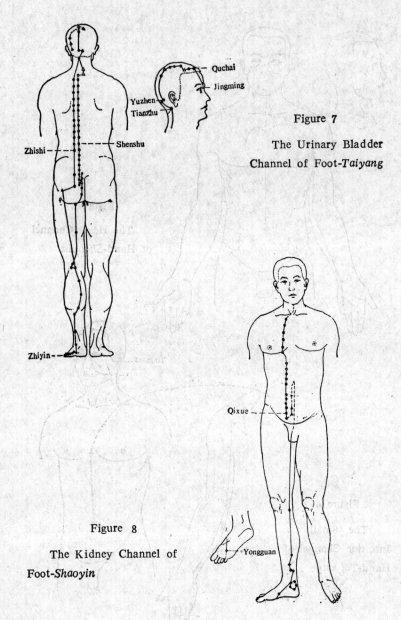

Quchai

Jingming

Yuzhen

Tianzhu

Zhishi —————— Shenshu

Zhiyin —

Qixue —

Yongguan —

Figure 7

The Urinary Bladder
Channel of Foot-*Taiyang*

Figure 8

The Kidney Channel of
Foot-*Shaoyin*

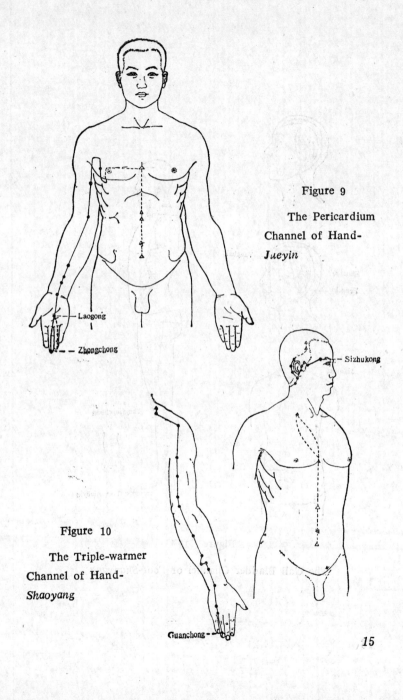

Figure 9

The Pericardium
Channel of Hand-
Jueyin

Laogong

Zhongchong

Sizhukong

Figure 10

The Triple-warmer
Channel of Hand-
Shaoyang

Guanchong

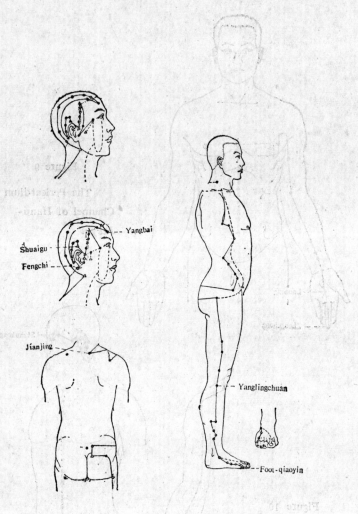

Figure 11

The Gall Bladder Channel of Foot-*Shaoyang*

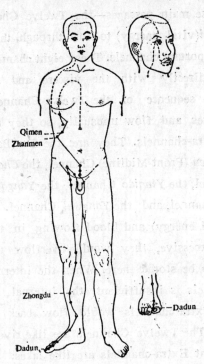

Qimen
Zhanmen

Zhongdu

Dadun

Dadun

Figure 12

The Liver Channel of
the Foot-*Jueyin*

Table 2.

Table 2

superficies of three *yang* (hollow organs)			interior of three *yin* (solid organs)
(2) Hand-*Yangming*	Large Intestine	←— lung ←—	(1) Hand-*Taiyin*
(3) Foot-*Yangming*	Stomach	—→spleen	(4) Foot-*Taiyin*
(6) Hand-*Taiyin*	Small Intestine	←—heart	(5) Hand-*Shaoyin*
(7) Foot-*Taiyin*	Urinary Bladder	—→kidney	(8) Foot-*Shaoyin*
(10) Hand-*Shaoyang*	Three-warmer	←—pericardium	(9) Hand-*Jueyin*
(11) Foot-*Shaoyang*	Gall Bladder—	—→liver	(12) Foot-*Jueyin*

17

In addition to these main passages—the Twelve Channels for the internal *Qi*(vital energy) to flow through, there are still eight other important channels. These eight channels do not communicate directly with the viscera and are not restricted by the sequence of the Twelve Channels. They take special routes and flow unusually, so they are called The Eight Extra-channels. They are: the *Du* (Back Midline) Channel, the *Ren* (Front Midline) Channel, the *Chong* Channel, the *Dai* Channel, the *Yinqiao* Channel, the *Yangqiao* Channel, the *Yinwei* Channel, and the *Yangwei* Channel.

When the *Qi* (vital energy) and blood flowing in the Twelve Channels are excessive, they would overflow the Eight Extra-channels to be stored there. When the internal *Qi* in the twelve channels is insufficient, the internal *Qi* stored in The Eight Extra-channels would flow back to The Twelve Channels. The Twelve Channels are like rivers and canals and the Eight Extra-channels are like lakes. So the function of the Eight Extra-channels is to maintain and to regulate The Twelve Channels. But The Eight Extra-channels have their own routes to take (see Figures 13— 20) and the internal *Qi* stored in them could warm the body organs internally and moisten the body surface, externally.

Any obstruction of the Twelve Channels or Eight Extra-channels could cause various kinds of related effects. In Chinese traditional medicine, this is described as "obstruction going before pain".

2. Promoting the Flowing of Internal *Qi* (vital energy)
   and Dredging the Channels and Collaterals

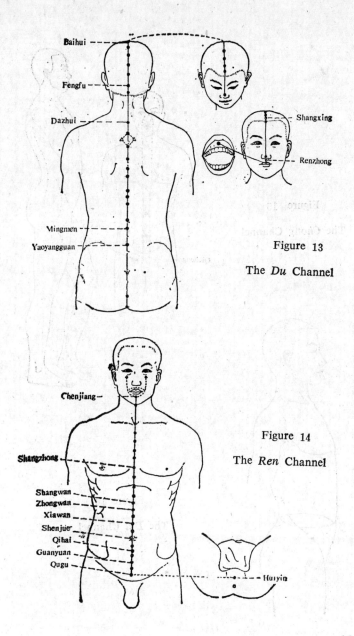

Baihui

Fengfu

Dazhui

Shangxing

Renzhong

Mingmen

Yaoyangguan

Figure 13

The *Du* Channel

Chenjiang

Shanzhong

Figure 14

The *Ren* Channel

Shangwan
Zhongwan
Xiawan
Shenjue
Qihai
Guanyuan
Qugu

Huiyin

19

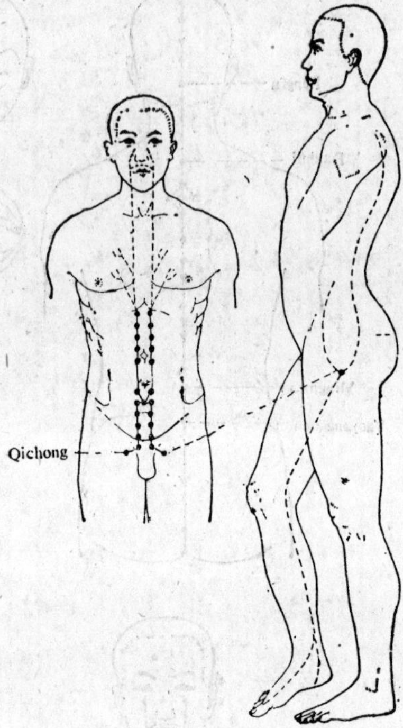

Figure 15

The *Chong* Channel

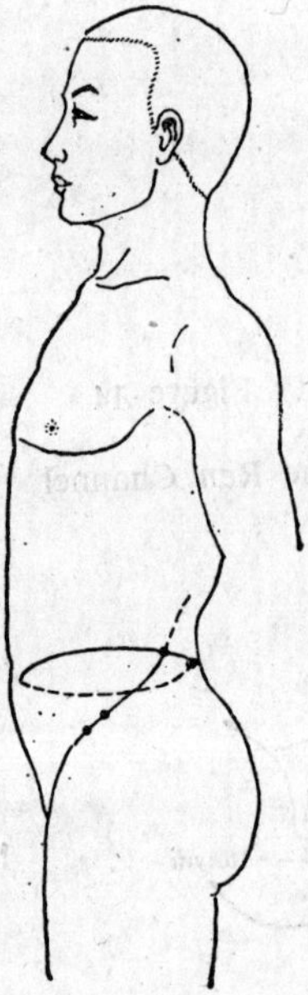

Qichong

Figure 16

The *Dai* Channel

Figure 17

The *Yangqiao* Channel

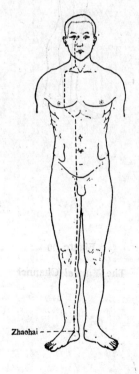

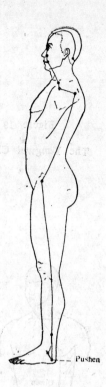

Pushen

Zhaohai

Figure 18

The *Yinqiao* Channel

21

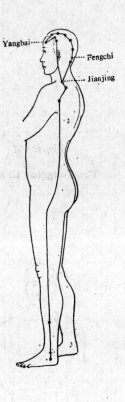

Figure 19

The *Yangwei* Channel

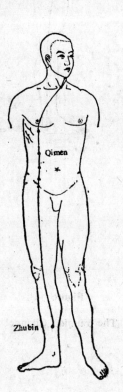

Figure 20

The *Yinwei* Channel

It is the human body's function and a natural and normal phenomenon that the internal *Qi* flows through the channels and collaterals. When the channels and collaterals in an individual's body are obstructed, the man will be sick. When a man is sick, the channels and collaterals in his body must be dredged, through a certain kind of force. Medicine, acupuncture and massage are therapies used as external force to dredge the channels and collaterals. Self-controlled *Qigong* therapy is used to dredge the channels and collaterals through relying on one's own force so that diseases can be treated.

In a chapter of "Familiar Conversation of *Nei Jing*, the Yellow Emperor's Canon of Internal Medicine" it says: "When the mind is quiescent and void, true *Qi* will be at your command. If one keeps a sound mind, his danger of disease will turn to safety." So the source of true *Qi* is closely related to the quiescence and emptying of the mind, which, in terms of *Qigong*, means "to be relaxed, quiescent and natural". To explicate it in the theory of modern medicine, this would put the cerebral cortex into a special inhibitory state, bring the regulating function of the central nervous system into play and improve and adjust the disorderly conditions of the nervous system so as to bring back to normal the functional and organic lesions caused by disturbance of the nervous system.

Thus it can be seen that a quiet mind is naturally the first precondition in promoting the flowing of internal *Qi*.

In the same chapter it also says, "If you take the whole world in your heart, have a good command of *yin* and

23

yang, breathe the essential *Qi* and keep a sound mind quiescently, your muscles will function smoothly and you will live as long as the earth exists."

The smooth functioning of the muscle means the recovery of health and the restoration of the original vitality. "To keep a sound mind" means to keep the mind in a quiescent state. To strengthen the internal *Qi* means to inhale essentail *Qi* and fresh air through breathing, that is, to enrich the postnatal *Qi* and augment the prenatal *Qi* with heavenly *Qi*. When the true *Qi* in prenatal *Qi* is adequate, the passage will be free from obstruction.

In another chapter of *Nei Jing* called "On Differential Proper Therapies" it also says, "To treat this disease ... *daoyin* and *anqiao* are appropriate."

Daoyin and *anqiao* are two different names given to *Qigong* in ancient times. *Daoyin* includes the mental *daoyin*, the breathing *daoyin* and the configuration (postural) *daoyin*. *Qiao* (in *anqiao*) means 'to lift up' i.e., 'to walk with the toes raised'; *an* (in *anqiao*) has two meanings: massage and the up-and-down movement of the wrists—a sort of empty massage. *Anqiao* refers to the methods of the configuration (postural) *daoyin*. The postures and movements in *Qigong* are different from those in other exercises, but the difference only lies in their intensities. So long as the exercise functions, it will benefit the acceleration of metabolism, the absorption and utilization of nutrition, the strengthening of health, and moreover, the flowing of true *Qi*.

To smoothen the channels and collaterals by means of

Qigong is a method as well as a purpose, because when the channels and collaterals are functioning smoothly, a person can possibly recover from his disease. As a result, it has the effect of preventing diseases and strengthening the health and finally in prolonging life.

One of the most important principles of the Chinese traditional medicine is to start with the body as a whole, to regulate the general system and diagnose and treat on the basis of an overall analysis of the illness and of the patient's condition; inflexible symptomatic treatment is discouraged. This principle also fits the case of *Qigong*. In the case of treating diseases with *Qigong*, the gerneral method is to start with a view to all the channels and collaterals, the solid and hollow organs and the internal *Qi*; it is a method to effect a permanent cure. However there also exist other methods of exercise used to treat diseases symptomatically. These include strengthening the connection between the channels and collaterals in the course of effecting permanent cures, in accordance with China's traditional medicine, and diagnosing and treating on the basis of overall analysis of the illness and the patient's condition. Beginners should not be too anxious to learn these symptomatic methods. Instead, they should follow the usual practice. And when the general condition is improved and the true *Qi* is adequate, it will be beneficial to learn some symptomatic methods so as to achieve the effect of protecting the health, and of casting away the disease.

3. Analysis of the Causes of Chronic Diseases

The China's traditional medicine summarizes the causes of the diseases of man as two: the interal and the external.

The internal cause of disease usually refers to the seven emotions that lead to diseases: joy, anger, grief, over-thinking, sadness, fear and terror. These emotional activities are physiological reactions to the external environment. Any emotional stress of excitement or inhibition would damage the viscera and cause visceral diseases. For example, sudden anger may lead to the disorder of liver; an excess of joy may lead to the disorder of heart; grief and over-thinking may lead to the disorder of spleen; sadness may lead to the disorder of lung; terror may lead to the disorder of kidney.Because the heart stores the spirit, all of them are related to the heart.

The diseases caused by the abnormality of the seven emotions are mainly reflected in organic changes. For example, anger causes Qi of the liver to go perversely upward and, as a result, stagnated anger may go upward to attack the mind and cause mental diseases; over-thinking may lead to the depression of Qi and obstruct the flow of Qi and finally the disorder of spleen and stomach occurs; sadness may lead to the consumption of Qi. Mental distress is caused by the disorder of lung; one may be confronted with sudden terror, and terror may lead to the abnormal descending of Qi which leads to the disorder of kidney and causes incontinence; fear may lead to the disorder of Qi, and may disturb the mind and the emotions, thus causing palpitation; excess of joy may lead to the slow flow of Qi and short-ness of breath occurs. Besides, emotional depression may obstruct the functional activities of *Qi* and stagnation may cause "fire", called the 'fire-syndrome caused by the disorders of the five emotions'. The 'fire-syndrome' may burn the fluid of the specific organ and cause the flaming-up of deficiency-fire (asthenic fire).

Modern medicine holds that 50—80% of the diseases are caused by nervousness, e.g. cancer, pulmonary diseases, heptic diseases, hypertension, cardiac diseases, ulcers etc.

The external cause of disease usually refers to the six kinds of weather changes of the four seasons such as wind, cold, summer-heat, wetness, dryness and fire—the six kinds of natural factors for short. These six kinds of natural factors function to promote the growth and development of all things on earth and are a condition on which man relies for his existence. However, if the weather changes excessively and abnormally, illnesses will occur. These abnormal weather factors that cause diseases are called 'six evils'. Of course, it is through the functioning of the human body that the six natural factors cause diseases. So it is directly proportional to the human body's adaptability and resistance (immunocompetence).

Of course, the external causes of diseases are not limited to the abnormal changes of weather. They also include some infectious pathogenic factors. But these infectious pathogenic factors are called 'the malicious natural factors' which are closely related with the 'six evils'. Therefore the 'six evils' not only affect the health of man, but also impact the formation and spreading of the 'malicious natural factors'.

27

4. Exploring the Mechanism of *Qigong* Therapy

Modern science has done a great deal of research on the medical theory of *Qigong*, which shares approximately our *Qigong* theory in three aspects:

Flaccid Reaction: According to his research Dr. Benson, an American expert, believes *Qigong* exercises may put the functions of the human body into the state of 'flaccid reaction'. The epidemiological theory on hypertension holds that the tension state may influence some physiological parameter. Environmental pressure causes the body to make some continuous adjustments. And therefore the so-called "stress response" (emergence reaction) occurs. As a result, the secretion of catecholamine increases; the blood in the skeletal muscles circulates more rapidly; the blood pressure rises accompanied by rapid heart-beat and breath. But the effect of 'flaccid reaction' is just the opposite. It weakens the activity of the sympathetic nervous system. The content of lactic acid in the arteries decreases and the metabolic rate drops; the activity of DBH in the plasma weakens and the activity of renin lessens.

'Systematization of Brain Cells': According to his study of ECG, Wallace explicates that the ECG of an ordinary person taken when conscious shows many high-frequency low negative waves with poor synchronism. But the ECG of a good *Qigong* practitioner shows many low-frequency positive waves, which is synchronic and three times higher than that of an ordinary person. This demonstrates that *Qigong* exercise can help systematize the electric activity of the

brain cells of the cerebral cortex. So the function of the brain is increased.

Preventing Disease and Prolonging Life: Qigong exercise can cause changes of central mediators (transmitters) and of the endocrine secretion. After the exercise, the density of prolactin in the plasma increases, which means the activity of dopamine as central mediators decreases, so it gives a sense of relaxation and calmness. Moreover, after the exercise, the secretion of cortin drops about 50%, which means the slowing-down of the aging process and enhancement of the functions of the immune system. So *Qigong* therapy has the effect of prolonging life and preventing diseases.

Theory:

(1) The Relaxed and Quiescent *Qigong* exercise can put the cerebral cortex into a 'special, protective, inhibitory state' and brings into play the inherent function of the cerebral cortex that regulates and repairs the viscera.

(2) Through regulating breath, it regulates the function of the vegetative nervous system. So the diseases caused by the disorder of the vegetative nervous system such as hypertension, gastric ulcer, neuroasthenia are repaired and regulated. Through the rising, descending, opening and closing patterns of breathing, it can also bring down the internal secretion, lower the quantity of cholesterol so as to treat cardiovascular diseases.

(3) Through regulating the mind and breath, it can improve the foci caused by pathologic reflex so as to treat various chronic diseases such as diseases of the heart, liver,

29

lung, spleen, neuroses and cancer.

(4) Through its dual nature of motivity and quiescence, *Qigong* exercise can increase the secretion of bile so as to enhance the digestive function.

The general principle is to invigorate the flow of internal *Qi* (vital energy) through *Qigong* exercise. When his inborn *Qi* is adequate, he will be free from the attack of all external noxious factors. The adequate *Qi* and smooth circulation of blood can regulate the *yin* and *yang* of the human body and invigorate and dredge the flow of essential *Qi*.

II. Some Characteristics of Self-Controlled *Qigong* Therapy

Self-controlled *Qigong* therapy has the following three aspects of chatacteristics:

(1) The inhaling of a large amount of fresh air provides the body with adequate oxygen. Therefore, blood circulation is intensified, physiological function regulated, immunocompetence enhanced and the health strengthened. This is one of the basic points of self-controlled *Qigong* therapy. As to how to inhale and exhale, it will be explained in detail in the starting posture of *Qigong* exercise and in detail in The Three Open-and-Close Form and in The Breath-Regulating and *Qi*-Reenforcing Pattern.

(2) To apply self-controlled *Qigong* therapy, it is required to carry out various kinds of breathing training exercises by using different body positions under the conditions of relaxation and quiescence. In the course of postural and

breathing training, the point is 'to promote quiescence with motion', 'to seek motion through quiescence' 'taking both motion and quiescence into consideration'. The cerebral cortex is put into a rest state so as to regulate the central nervous system and effect treatment. 'To promote quiescence with motion' means to let the central nervous system have a rest in a state of low frequency oscillation. 'To seek motion through quiescence' means that under the precondition of quiescence you make a few movements clear-mindedly to promote the smooth flow of internal Qi (vital energy) and dredge the channels and collaterals. This feature works to promote the flow of internal Qi with external movements and the flow of internal Qi is acquired under the precondition of quiescence. That is, with relaxation, concentration of the mind and the downward movement of the internal Qi from the center of the channel-collaternal system, automatic (internal) motivity is produced. So the medical effect of the self-controlled $Qigong$ therapy can be demonstrated in a short period of time.

(3) The self-controlled $Qigong$ therapy can be easily accepted. It possesses motivity, quiescence and a flexible variety of exercise patterns. It's easy to perform and can also be taken by patients. It's very effective, too. That's why it is liked so much by the boad masses of people.

31

Chapter 2
The *Daoyin* Function of Some Basic Postures

The basic poses of *Qigong* training play an important role in the self-controlled *Qigong* therapy. The success in *Qigong* training is directly related with the correctness of body positions. A correct body position is the impetus for training as well as training technique that works through the whole course. It includes three aspects: regulating the heart, regulating the breath and regulating the physical body.

Regulating the heart means regulating the mind. A sound mind leads to downward flow of *Qi*, which effects sound pulse conditions (diastole of blood vessels) and promotes good health. In other words, when the posture is correct, *Qi* will flow freely, i.e., *Qi* flows in accordance with the changes of body positions. *Qi* also directs the circulation of blood. That is why it is called "the commander of blood"; *Qi* is also dominated by the heart and mind, so it's also said that "the mind is the commander of *Qi*". Therefore, the three aspects, regulating the heart, regulating breath and regulating the physical body form an inseparable whole unit.

The starting forms of self-controlled *Qigong* therapy are classified into three: The Relaxed and Quiescent Form in

Standing Pose, the Three Slow Exhaling and Inhaling Form and the Three Open-and-Close Form. The ending forms are the same as the starting ones, but the sequence is reversed. It is believed that these three forms of technique make up the starting and ending poses of various styles of *Qigong* exercise of the self-controlled *Qigong* therapy. The function of the starting pose is to calm down the heart so as to have a peaceful mind. When the *Qi* flows freely, one is ready for the next step of exercise. The function of the ending poses is to bring the *Qi* back to *Dantian*. The effect of nourishing the *Qi* is achieved in the course of bringing the *Qi* back and concentrating the mind.

I . Function of the Relaxed and Quiescent Form in Standing Pose

The Relaxed and Quiescent Form in Standing Pose includes 18 steps of action: standing on flat feet, knee-bending, hip-relaxing, crotch-rounding, anus-lifting, stomach-pulling in, waist-relaxing, chest-tucking in, back-stretching, shoulder-drooping, elbow-dropping armpit-hollowing, wrist-relaxing, head-suspending, cheek-hooking, eye-shutting, lip-closing and tongue touching the upper teeth ridge. The specific requirement of each step is as follows:

Standing on flat feet: Stand with feet flat and set them apart as wide as the two shoulders with the weight evenly on two feet out bear no pressure on the waist and the coccyx, thus paving the way for relaxing the waist.

Knee-bending: The knee-joint is the main joint for a sufficient amount of *Qi* and blood to pass through. A relaxed

33

knee-joint that is free from rigidity will be favourable for the *Qi* and blood to flow and meanwhile making it easy for hip-relaxing and crotch-rounding as well as preparing for waist-relaxing.

Hip-relaxing: When the hip-joints are relaxed, the lower limbs will be able to move freely.

Crotch-rounding: The first step in crotch-rounding is to set the knees apart and the second step is to bring them together, which is combined with hip-relaxing. Meanwhile the knee-caps are lifted, so a sense of lightness is felt in the lower limbs. The third step is to suspend the crotch— to lift the perineum and the anus slightly. The function of crotch-rounding is to keep the perineum free from pressure and yet not open. That the perineum is free from pressure ensures better functional activities of the *Qi* and its not being open is for the "lower door" to remain closed permanently (avoiding leakage of vital energy).

Anus-lifting: The same as above.

Stomach-pulling-in: This is meant to pull in the abdomen above the pubic bone, avoiding tension of the abdominal muscles. Stomach-pulling-in helps to restrain the primordial *Qi*, which increases the internal pressure and promotes the flow of internal *Qi* throughout the whole body.

Waist-relaxing: "If the waist is not relaxed, the *Qi* can not sink back to *Dantian*." The basic action of waist-relaxing is to relax the hips and bend the knees. When the waist is relaxed, the spine will stand upright and remain downward relaxed. The specific actions are as follows: Lift both shoulders and relax them downward immediately; give a deep breathing-out and now the waist is relaxed. Waist-relaxing is the keypoint of relaxation. To achieve genuine waist-relaxation, one has to relax and move the sacral bone. But the sacral bone is a kind of pseudoarthrosis. An ordinary person can not move it. Only when a woman is pregnant, can this bone become loose and elastic. However, a regular *Qigong* performer may have sufficient primordial *Qi* to thrust it open. When this pseudoarthrosis is opened, the space of *Dantian* will be expanded and the store of primordial *Qi* will be enlarged. This is a good preparation for the activation of joints afterwards.

Chest-tucking-in: This means an intentional tucking-in of the chest. It does not indicate the inward thrust of shoulders, nor does it suggest the intentional closure of the thoracic cavity. It refers to the relaxation of the chest. The intentional tucking-in of the vertebrae area requires the outward opening of the ribs. The unification of the outward opening and the inward tucking helps to relax the thoracic cavity, thus providing a more spacious thoracic cavity and avoiding tension of the thoracic muscles.

Back-stretching: To stretch the back means to let the vertebrae stand upright in the middle. The key point in back-stretching is to droop the shoulders. The two shoulders drop evenly and the lumbar vertebrae straighten out.

The function of chest-tucking-in and back-stretching is to calm the heart and lung. The heart and the lung are located inside the chest. The heart controls mental and emotional activities and also directs blood circulation. When the thoracic cavity is spacious and the back stands upright, the heart and mind will be calm, and the lung will be clear and free from heat. Chest-tucking-in and back-stretching make the chest and back relaxed, which is favourable for the *Ren* Channel and the *Du* Channel to communicate with each other.

Shoulder-drooping: Relax the shoulder-joints and let them droop naturally and the shoulders and neck will be relaxed.

Elbow-dropping: It is necesary to bend the elbow slightly before it is dropped. The dropping sensation is felt at the elbow point. The dropping requires suspending, or there is a sensation of compression at the shoulder and the elbow.

"Armpit-hollowing": To droop the shoulders, it is necessary to "hollow" the armpits. To achieve this, the keypoint is to move the two elbows exteriorly to the left and right. Attention should be paid to avoiding sloping or square shoulders. When the armpits are maintained hollow, the *Qi* and blood in the upper limbs will flow freely.

Wrist-relaxing: This includes wrist relaxation, palm hollowing and comfortable closure of the fingers. Wrist relaxation makes the *Shu* Point in the wrist communicate with the fingers.

Palm-hollowing and finger-closing suggest natural stretching and curving. Rigidity and purposeful bending should be avoided. Palm-hollowing and finger-closing prevent the *Qi* from diffusing. The above-mentioned four items help regulate the six channels—the three *yang* channels of hand and the three *yin* channels of hand, so the *Qi* and blood can flow freely, which effects a sensation of lightness and ease in the upper limbs. It is well-known that the 'hand' plays a decisive role in the evolutionary history of man. The evolution of the hand promoted the development of the brain and finally man rose above the animal kingdom. The mutual influences of the hand and the brain incessantly develop. With the incessant development of the mutual influence and mutual promotion of the hand and the brain the connection between the two became ever closer. The saying "hand is the flag" in *Qigong* theory also helps explain the leading function of the hand. Some scientific experiments indicate that there is a clear demonstration of the impact of mental activities on the bioelectricity of the hand.

Head-suspending: Keep the head as if it were suspended. Suspension produces vacancy. When suspended, the head must be kept in the middle and absolutely upright. This helps set the whole body in the upright position. An upright and vacant head is not only the key point in setting the whole body in an upright position, but also in directing the *Qi* and blood to flow upward so as to nourish the brain and mind. Therefore, the mechanism of the "spirit", which controls all the physical activities, will be reinforced while the essence of life, the *Qi* and the spirit will be invigorated.

Cheek-hooking: This means to tuck in the chin. Only when the chin is tucked in, can the *Baihui* Point on the head be uprightly suspended and the respiration kept free.

Eye-shutting: It is required that the eyes are closed as if curtains were drawn. The upper eyelids droop natually, but not tightly shut. Tight shutting would cause tension in the upper and lower eye-lids. Then the eyelids are gently closed, the vision is held back, which helps calm the soul and spirit. The eyes look into the distance horizontally. This can regulate the venous pressure in the cranial cavity.

Lip-closing: To have the lips and teeth gently closed with the molars in the biting position is the method to enhance the *yang* in *Qigong* exercise. Closed lips prevent the internal *Qi* from flowing out.

The Tongue Touching the Upper Palate: This in fact requires that the tongue touch the teeth ridge without force. One of its functions is to play the role of the *bridge of magpies* commonly known as *building a bridge*. The aim of *building a bridge* is to make the *Ren* Channel communicate with the *Du* Channel. The *Ren* Channel is responsible for all the *yin* channels. It starts from the *Baogong* (where the uterus is in women), turns upward at *Huiyin*, passes through *Guanyuan* and *Qihai* and finally reaches *Chengjiang*. The *Du* Channel governs all the *yang* channels. It also starts from the extreme lower part *Shu* Point, joins *Jili* and goes up to *Fengfu*, *Baihui* and then to the nose bridge by way of the forehead. When these two channels communicate with each other, there will be an exchange of *yin* and *yang*. This can eliminate diseases and prolong a person's life. One of the two communicated channels ends in the nose, the other ends in the mouth. The tongue links them up. That's why it is called *the bridge of magpies*. Besides, there are the points of *Jinzin*, *Yuye* and *Haiquan*; when the tongue touches the palate, saliva will be increased. The saliva contains many kinds of enzyme, which not only help digestion but also benefit physiology. It was called *god water* in our country in ancient times.

In the above-mentioned relaxation and standing that consist of 18 items, the main point in postural *daoyin* (guiding and inducing) is relaxing. And the aim of relaxing is to seek quiescence. Among other things, the general function is to guide the flow of *Qi* along the channels. This is the most important basic technique in *Qigong* training.

Ⅱ. **Function of the Three Deep Exhaling and Inhaling Form**

The Three Deep Exhaling and Inhaling Form is aimed at regulating the symptoms caused by the preponderance of *yang* and the deficiency of *yin*, which is characterized by sthenia-symptom in the upper part and asthenia in the lower, through deep, thin and even breathing exercise of *daoyin*. In terms of physiology, deep exhaling can stimulate the parasympathetic nerves. The excitatory parasympathetic nerves help promote the blood vessels to dilate and therefore have the function of bringing down blood pressure. Deep inhaling can stimulate the sympathetic nerves. The excitatory sympathetic nerves promote the blood vessels to contract and function to elevate blood pressure. The alternation between deep exhaling and inhaling produces the diastole and systole of the blood vessels and enhances the elasticity of their walls.

The alternation between deep exhaling and inhaling can also temper the excitation and inhibition of the sympathetic nerves and the parasypathetic nerves and therefore regulates the vegetative nerves. According to the analysis of the effects of *Qigong*, the descending mechanism in the three deep exhalings and inhalings is stronger than the ascending mechanism with all the postures downward. And the mental activities, as affected by the postures, are also generally downward. So it has a kind of downward *daoyin* function to the diseases caused by the preponderance of *yang*. Besides, as deep exhaling helps to keep the *yin* going downward and inhaling helps to keep the *yang* going upward, it also has the effect of propping up the *yang* and tranquilizing the mind.

Ⅱ. Function of the Three Open-and-Close Form

The term open-and-close refers to the opening and closing of the *Qi* guided by different postures. The opening of the *Qi* is guided by the outward movement of the hands and arms, and meanwhile in the mental activities there is also an opening or expanding intention in the abdomen. The closing of the *Qi* is guided by the simultaneous inward movement of the hands and arms toward the abdomen for a closing-up. The mind is also concentrated on the abdomen. This is in fact what is called abdominal breathing. The opening means exhaling, which makes the abdomen expand. The closing means inhaling, which makes the abdomen contract. The expansions and contractions of the abdomen result in the mental concentration on the abdomen. Actually the mind is focused on *Dantian*. *Dantian* is located at *Qihai* (the vital-energy sea) below the umbilicus. The nerves in this area are the neuroplex of *Taiyang* (major *yang*). If the mind is concentrated on *Dantian* for a long time, there would occur a *Qigong* reflex arc at the *Taiyang* neuroflex nerve endings around *Dantian*. So there forms a conditioned reflex that causes the *Taiyang* neuroflex to produce bioelectricity that spreads to the surroundings, impacts the small blood vessels to dilate, reduces the pressure of blood vessels and decreases the burden of the heart so as to improve blood circulation, i.e., improve the general nutritional condition and therefore the diseases caused by malnutrition can be treated.

Chapter 3
The *Daoyin* Function of the Breath-Regulating and *Qi*-Reenforcing Pattern

The function of the Breath-Regulating and *Qi*-Reenforcing Pattern is, through regulating the breath and breathing in the essence of vital energy (*Qi*), to invigorate vitality and make the blood and vital energy function well, so as to eliminate disease and promote longevity. In *The Formation of the Five Solid Organs, Familiar Conversation*, it says, "The vital energy is connected with the lung. The lung controls the vital energy. The natural vital energy outside

41

the human body is inhaled through the lung. The vital energy from the food inside the body goes up into the lung through the spleen-pulse. The two are combined and stored in the vital energy "sea" of the chest, which is called "initial energy." In *Evil Factors, Spiritual Pivot*, it says, "The initial energy is stored in the chest and exhaled through the throat. It passes through the heart-pulse to carry out breathing activities." So this *Qigong* pattern of regulating breath and reenforcing vital energy functions as the main method to regulate the channels of the lung and bring the function of the lung into full play.

The lung is closely related with the other organs. while the heart controls blood circulation, the lung controls the vital energy. The human body relies on the vital energy and blood to transport nourishment, maintain the functional activities of the various organs and the normal relationship among them. Although the circulation of blood is controlled by the heart, only when the lung-energy flows freely can the blood penetrate the heart-pulse and pass through the whole body.

The lung is also closely related with the spleen, the stomach, the kidney, the gate of life and the bladder. In *Special Theory on Channel System, Familiar Conversation*, it says, "Fluid is taken into the stomach. The vital energy diffuses and circulates up into the spleen. The spleen-energy spreads up to the lung. It dredges the water passage and flows down into the bladder" ... If the lung-energy fails to descend normally, it may rise adversely and causes dyspnea and cough.

If the fluid metabolism is affected, it may cause retention of fluid and retention of urine and edema occurs. The kidney plays a very important role in fluid metabolism. With the descent of the lung-energy, the fluid flows down into the kidney. The fluid that flows into the kidney is turbid fluid. The turbid part of the turbid fluid will be expelled out of the body through the bladder. The clear part of the turbid fluid will be changed into vital energy at "the triple warmer" and goes up to the lung, where it is circulated and changed into water and descends into the kidney. This circulation maintains the balance of the fluid metabolism of the body. The "gate of life" is also called the source of "the prime-minister fire" of "the triple warmer". Fire failure at "the triple warmer" will lead to the unsuccessful formation of vital energy. And blockage of water passage may cause edema, phlegm-retention diseases, dyspepsia, and dyspnea in the case of lung. Besides, there are other causes of dyspnea, e.g. failure of kidney-energy in aiding lung to regulate respiration and stasis of lung-energy caused by blockage of water passage. So in *Classic on Medical Problems* "the gate of life" is described as the "gate for respiration and source of the triple warmer."

"The gate of life" and the kidney rule over the innate qualities. (Some people say "the gate of life" is located to the right of the left kidney; others say it is between the two kidneys; still others say "the gate of life" has two aspects of function—the spleen-*yin* and the spleen-*yang*. The prenatal primordial energy needs to be continuously supplemented by postnatal energy. The postnatal heavenly energy and earthly energy (essential substance from cereals) rely on the smooth circulation of lung-energy. So regulating breath and strengthening the lung are to reenforce the prenatal energy, i.e., to greatly enhance the primordial energy. This *Qigong* technique functions to regulate vital energy and blood, tonify and nourish primordial energy. "When attacked by evil-factors, there must be a deficiency of vital energy." The asthenia-syndrome should be treated by therapy of invigoration. The sthenia-syndrome should be treated by purgation. Cancer and tumour both belong to sthenia-syndrome caused by long-term stagnation of vital energy and blood stasis. This technique will have a special effect if it is made, by changing the speed of *daoyin* technique, to function as a treatment of sthenia-syndrome as well as a reenforcement of primordial energy.

The basic principle of the Breath-Regulating and *Qi*-Reenforcing Pattern is to breathe in the heavenly and earthly healthy energy; to enrich the primordial energy by breathing in more and breathing out less. So the *daoyin* technique of breathing is mainly designed as 'two breathings-in with one breathing-out'. The blowing method of inhaling and exhaling through the nose is adopted because the nose is the orifice to the lung. In *Pulse-Style of Spiritual Pivot*, it says, "The lung-energy leads to the nose". A patient with lung-asthenia usually has a stuffy nose. If a patient with lung disease has rapid respiration, there may occur the symptom of fanning nostrils. So the blowing method designed to use the nasal cavity is aimed at strengthening the nose and opening the inhibited lung-energy.

The postural function of *daoyin* in regulating breath and reenforcing vital energy mainly relies on the movement of the hand and arm to the left and to the right so as to arouse and invigorate the vital energy circulating in the lung channel of hand *Taiyin* and the large intestine channel of hand *Yangming* (These two channels share a paired relationship). At the same time, it is required that the toes should be raised with the heel touching the ground to stimulate the *Yinqiao* channel and the *Yangqiao* channel and strengthen the working function of the physical body as well as the function of the kidney channel and the urinary bladder channel.

The Breath-Regulating and *Qi*-Reenforcing Pattern has 4 kinds of *daoyin* technique which have the following effects in addition to what is mentioned above:

Fixed-step Blowing Method: Move, by stepping out onto the right foot and then the left foot with the toes raised, for 9 times. Its main function is to quide the lung-energy to descend and lead "the prime-minister fire" from "the gate of life" to rise so as to warm the lung-energy.

The Kidney-Strengthening Method: This is the basic *Qigong* technique to regulate breath and reenforce the vital energy. Breathe in the essence of vital energy so as to reenforce the prenatal energy.

The Method to Strengthen the Lung, the Liver and the Spleen: On the basis of *the kidney-Strengthening Method*, let

45

the thumb and index-finger rub each other and make friction between the *Shaoshang* Point and the *Shaoyang* Point so as to invigorate the flow of the vital energy along the lung channel and the large intestine channel, which has a lung-strengthening function. When walking with the toes raised, let the big toe touch the ground so as to stimulate the *Yinbai* Point and the *Dadun* Point on the big toe and promote the internal energy to flow upward along the liver channel and the spleen channel. So the internal energy of these two channels can be reenforced and the liver and spleen strengthened.

The Heart-Strengthening Method: This method means to walk at a slightly slow speed. At the third step the middle finger of each hand touches the centre of the palm. Its function is to stimulate the *Zhongchong* Point so as to invigorate the flow of the internal energy along the pericardium channel.

Chapter 4
The *Daoyin* Function of The Toe–Raised Transport and Conversion Pattern

The Toe-Raised Transport and Conversion Pattern of *Qigong* is the essential technique of the self-controlled

Qigong therapy. It consists of three items: a) the rising, falling, opening and closing of the three *Dantians* b) toe-raised slow walking and inducing the vital energy to come back to *Dantian* and c) kneading the abdomen.

Ⅰ. Function of The Open-and-Close Method at the Three *Dantians*

The technique of this method is to open and close once at each of the three points: the Upper *Dantian—Yintang*, the Middle *Dantian—Qihai*, and the Lower *Dantian—Huiyin*.

The *daoyin* function of the opening and closing of the Upper *Dantian* is to let the lucid *yang* ascend to the upper orifices, act on the body surface and strengthen the four extremities. When the lucid *yang* moves upwards, it is clear and quiet and helps to tranquilize the mind. To act on the body surface means to use body respiration to *inhale heavenly energy* so as to *have a sound mind* and to regulate the body and the four limbs so as to make the tendons flexible. "When the body is open, the evil will be expelled". "Now that the body surface is free from evil-factors, it is better to have it closed."

The aim of opening and closing the Middle *Dantian* and Lower *Dantian* is to make the turbid-*yin* descend and its significance is to store the essence of vital energy. The part below the waist belongs to *yin*. The kidney is not the only organ to store the essence of vital energy. All the five solid organs store it. So the saying goes, "The *yin* is what stores extremely well the essence of vital energy. And the *yang* is what guards against the exogenous evils and protects the body." "Adequate *yin* leads to the formation of *yang* and adequate *yang* leads to the strengthening of *yin*." When the *yin* and *yang* are in balance, "the tendons and pulse will be in harmony; the bone structure will be solid and the blood and vital energy will circulate freely."

The application of the theory of China's traditional medicine to *Qigong* can be presented in four words in terms of *daoyin* technique: *rise, fall, open* and *close. Rise* leads to the ascending of the vital energy, *fall* its descending, *open* its spreading and *close* its restraining. In the course of ascending, descending spreading and restraining, the vital energy can be regulated, smoothened, reenforced and suplemented. Therefore, to a person with hyperactive ascending vital energy (e.g. hypertension), he should hold his hands with the palms downward and the two hands move from the two sides of the body quickly upward. when the hands move downward, the two middle fingertips touch each other with the palms facing downward and move slowly downward along the front of the body so as to guide and induce the mechanism of the vital energy to descend. A person with *yin* and *yang* unbalanced (e.g. neurasthenia) should have his palms facing the body or facing upward when moving upward, and facing downward when moving downward to move with a similar speed so as to guide and induce the lucid *yang* to ascend, the turbid *yin* to descend and therefore the *yin* and *yang* are balanced. A person with deficiency of descending vital energy (e.g. prolapse of viscera) should, when moving up the hands, have his palms face upward and rise

48

slowly close to the body and, when moving them down, get away quickly from the body so as to avoid an excessive downward flow as a result of *daoyin*, but to effect an upward flow. In short, the opening and closing of the three *Dantians* can regulate the overabundance-syndrome and the asthenia-syndrome caused by the unbalance between the upper and the lower, and the interior and the exterior.

It is required that the opening and closing at the three *Dantians* should be performed once facing each of the four directions in the sequence of east, north, west and south and once again in the sequence of south, west, north and east, because although the internal energy flows inside the human body, like the atmosphere of nature, in a very complicated way, it also has a certain regularity.

Early in the morning the sun rises in the eastern sky. The energy (*Qi*) from the east, which is called *Shaoyang*, is the energy that controls birth. At noon time, the sun shines in the south. The energy from the south, which is called *Laoyang*, is the energy that controls development. In the afternoon, the sun turns to the west. The energy from the west, which is called *Shaoyin*, is the energy that controls astringency. In the evening, the sun sets in the north. The energy from the north, which is called *Laoyin*, is the energy that controls storage. The energy inside the human body flows in a similar way as the great nature. Liver-energy belongs to *Shaoyang*—the energy from the east that controls birth. Heart-energy belongs to *Laoyang*—energy from the south that controls development. Lung-energy belongs to

Shaoyin—the energy from the west that controls astringency. Kidney-energy belongs to *Laoyin*—the energy from the north that controls storage. These energies exchange incessantly. For example, the rapid rising of the heart-energy needs to be inhibited by the kidney-energy which has a powerful downward pulling function. The excessive tendency of the kidney-energy to constrict and descend also needs to be eased by a force which rises rapidly. So in the convection, these energies inhibit each other, encourage each other and foster each other so as to avoid sthenia phenomena such as too much downward pressure, cold, heat and hyperactivity. According to their different locations, heart-energy is at the top; kidney-energy is at the bottom; liver-energy is on the left; lung-energy is on the right. It is necessary for the human body to have some exchange of internal energies between the upper and the lower parts, and between the left and right sides. The internal energies have different characteristics. Heart-energy is like fire; kidney-energy is like water; liver-energy is like wood and lung-energy is like gold. Inside the human body it is necessary for the water and fire to counter-act each other and for the gold and wood to exchange and blend. Yet, any uninterrupted exchange either between the upper and the lower, between the left and the right or between the gold and the wood, requires some vital energy that flows continuously, evenly and has the function of transportation and conversion. And this vital energy is the spleen-energy in the human body. Spleen-energy is free from deviation to wrong directions. It not only can take in various kinds of vital energies, but also can send them out, after converting them, so as to enable them to foster each other, utilize each other and restrain each other; the *yin*-energy is maintained mild and the *yang*-energy is consolidated. So the "spirit", which commands vital activities, and the "essence", which sustains the substances for vital activities, can be kept in a normal and stable state.

II. Function of the Toe-Raised Slow-Walking Method

The purpose to raise the toes is to invigorate the *Yinxiao* Channel and the *Yangqiao* Channel. The function of toe-raising has been explained previously in the Breath-Regulating and *Qi*-Reenforcing Pattern. The following passage will deal with the function of Toe-Raised Slow Walking. The necessity to walk slowly when toes are raised is decided by the mild nature of the spleen. The spleen is located inside the abdomen. Its channels are connected with the stomach and it shares a paired relationship with the stomach. The spleen has the physiological function of converting and transporting nutrition, benefiting vital energy, controlling blood and dissipating phlegm. It is also responsible for the growth of muscles and for the activities of the extremities. So in ancient times, the spleen and stomach were called "source of postnatal energy". As the spleen is responsible for the activity of the extremities, the movement of the four limbs also has the function to strengthen the spleen. So "toe-raised walking" and "hand-swaying" have been adopted for the style and posture of this *Qigong* training.

Patients with spleen trouble usually have symptoms such as dyspepsia, watery diarrhea, flaccidity of the four limbs, muscular emaciation and general hypofunction. The commonly known hematochezia (bloody stool) and prolonged menorrhagia are actually caused by deficiency of spleen-energy when the kidney loses its control.

Toe-raised slow-walking not only strengthens the transporting and converting function of the spleen with postural *daoyin*, but also plays an important role in mental *daoyin*. The spleen is closely related with all the solid and hollow organs. Its relationship with the heart is even closer. when the heart-channels are vigorous, the spleen-channels will function normally and more vigorously. The heart controls the mental and the emotional activities. So mental *daoyin* plays a more important role in the Toe-Raised Transport and Conversion Pattern of *Qigong* exercise.

Ⅱ. **Function of Bringing the Vital Energy Back to *Dantian* and Kneading the Abdomen**

Bringing the vital energy back to *Dantian* actually includes two forms of *Qigong* exercise—The Open-and-Close at the Two *Dantians* (i.e. the open-and-close at the Upper *Dantian* and the Middle *Dantian*) and Kneading the Abdomen.

1. Function of the Open-and-Close at the Two *Dantians*

The open-and-close at the two *Dantians* has a tranquilizing function like that of the open-and-close at the three *Dantians*. When you are in quiescence and relaxation, if you are disturbed by something in the surroundings, you can do

52

open-and-close at the two *Dantians* a few times and your mind will be tranquilized. The open-and-close at the Middle *Dantian* has the function to secure the solid and hollow organs and to bring the vital energy back to *Dantian*.

2. Function of Kneading the Abdomen

To knead the abdomen 36 times clockwise and 24 times anti-clockwise not only coincides with the figure of the functional activities of the vital energy, but also fits the method to bring the vital energy back to *Dantian*.

Ⅳ. Exploration of the Mechanism of the Toe-Raised Transport and Conversion Pattern

To explore *Qigong* in terms of modern physiology, the mechanism of the Toe-Raised Transport and Conversion Pattern is summarised as follows:

1. Mechanism of the Mental *Daoyin*

When the mind is concentrated on *Qihai* (sea of vital energy), the local area of skin and the neuroplex of *Tai-yang* beneath it will be stimulated and produce the function of conditioned reflex. Physiologically, *Qihai* is connected with the vegetative nerves, the sympathetic nerves and para-sympathetic nerves on all the viscera such as the kidney, the pancreas, the intestines, the liver, the spleen, the stomach and the medullary nucleus. The receptors of these nerves transmit to the nerve centre and then to the effectors. The effectors regualate the blood pressure and substance metabo-lism, promoting the reaction of excretion and assimilation. This makes the cerebral cortex participate in the conditioned reflex passively. The existing pathological reflex arc is changed to *Qigong* reflex arc, i.e. the normal physiological reflex arc. This is the physiological function of mental *daoyin*.

2. Mechanism of Breathing *Daoyin*

In the deep exhaling and inhaling of the open-and-close, a lot of carbon dioxide is expelled through the deep exhaling, which excites the parasympathetic nerves and makes the capillaries at the abdomen dilate, while through the inhaling a lot of oxygen is taken in, which excites the sympathetic nerve, makes the blood vessels contract and causes the blood pressure to rise. These repeated alternations can promote blood circulation and strengthen the contracting ability of the heart so as to improve or cure heart trouble.

3. Mechanism of the Postural *Daoyin*

When the body is in motion, as a result of the contraction, squeezing and pressing of the bones and muscles, the blood in the veins can not flow back after it goes up and passes the valves. Blood can only be supplied by the capillaries. This unique physiological function is called "the pump function of the muscles". The open-and-close with the rising and falling movements and the swaying of the four limbs all can promote the "pump function of the muscles". The Toe-Raised Transport and Conversion Pattern is designed to employ this function. The bending and leaning of the upper part of the body, the squatting and crouching with the lower limbs as well as the walking with alternate weighty and weightless steps can all promote "the pump function of the muscles" and promote backflow of the blood in the veins so as to invigorate physiological function.

54

Chapter 5
Function of Mental *Daoyin*
(Method to Regulate the Heart)

To regulate the heart is in fact to regulate the mind—that is, to regulate the cerebral cortex so as to recover the unbalanced part of the cerebral cortex.

Ⅰ. **Function of Regulating the Heart—to Reenforce the Five Solid Organs**

The agitation of the heart can cause the agitation of all the five solid organs. Only under the unified command of the heart, can the five solid organs and six hollow organs support each other and cooperate to maintain normal vital activities.

Thoughts and mental activities are reflexes of the brain and cerebral cortex. If the mind is agitated or depressed for a long time, it will cause a long-term disorder to the whole nervous system and thus cause various kinds of chronic diseases. Take hypertension for example, its mechanism is summarized as follows:

To carry on their activities, various kinds of cells and organs connect and cooperate with each other and inhibit each other through the adjustment of the nervous system. The nervous system is the system that takes the leading role

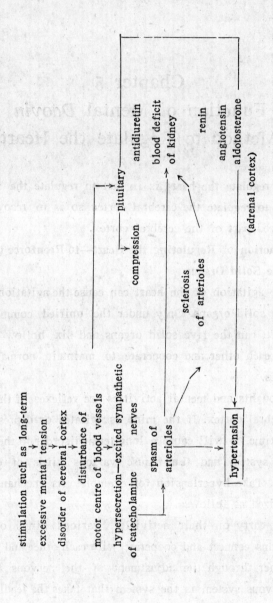

stimulation such as long-term
excessive mental tension
→ disorder of cerebral cortex
→ disturbance of
motor centre of blood vessels
→ hypersecretion—excited sympathetic
of catecholamine   nerves
→ spasm of
arterioles   → hypertension

sclerosis
of arterioles

pituitary → antidiuretin
→ blood deficit
of kidney

compression

renin
angiotensin
aldotosterone
(adrenal cortex)

in adjustment and regulation. It can recognize the environmental changes inside the physical body, control the activities of the body and its viscera, make them coordinate their activities with the whole body so as to maintain a dynamic equilibrium and therefore the unity of all functional activities and a relative stability of the internal environment.

The environmental changes outside the physical body can inevitably cause new contradictions inside the body, which leads to new imbalances. The nervous system can recognize the environmental changes outside the body and make the body adapt its activities to these changes so as to maintain a relative stability in the ever changing external environment.

So the function of the body is to obtain a unity of opposites between the internal and external environments under the leadership role of the nervous system.

Traditional medicine believes, The heart stores the spirit and controls mental and emotional activities. It is related with the spirit and emotion. Li Shizhen, a famous ancient Chinese doctor, said: "The brain is the supreme mental palace". When the heart has some functional disorder, mental and emotional activities will be out of control. The heart not only controls the spirit but also controls blood vessels. If the blood vessels do not function normally, emotional activities will also be out of control. On the other hand, blood circulation is, to an extent, influenced by emotions. This happens to be identical with the theory of modern medicine.

I. Function of Conditioned Reflex and Reflex Arc

The nerve reflex arc consists of five parts: the receptor, the afferent nerve, the nerve centre, the efferent nerve and the effector.

Reflex is divided into non-conditioned reflex and conditioned reflex.

Non-conditioned reflex refers to inherent, autonomic activities of the nerves such as sucking, saliva secretion, open-and-close of eyes and so on. These are man's instinctive activities.

Conditioned reflex is a more complicated formal reaction based on non-conditioned reflex. For example, "to quench one's thirst by thinking of plums" is to arouse the secretion of saliva through an imagined sour sensation.

II. Endocrines Influenced by Emotions and Mood

Emotions and mood can arouse nerve impulses. Nerve impulses involve the production of physiological and chemical substances. When a person is angry or terrified, adrenalin is produced to excite the sympathetic nerves. As a result, the secretion of saliva is decreased, the rate of respiration and heartbeat is increased in order to make the blood flow to the whole body. This is a protective reaction of the body. However, long-term continuous anger or terror will lead to the contraction of blood vessels, spasm or even sclerosis of the arterioles and an insufficient supply of blood. So gastric ulcer, gastroduadenal ulcer and hypertension are caused. Any disturbance of the endocrines will weaken the immunity (resistance) of the human body. According to China's statistics of esophagal cancer, patients with worry and anxiety as the causes make up 56% in Shanxi Province, 69% in Hebei Province and 64% in Shandong Province. About 52% of the patients had been badly upset half a year before they got sick.

From the above-mentioned analysis of the causes of diseases, it can been seen that chronic diseases are closely related to patients' emotions and moods. To treat such chronic diseases, it is necessary, first of all, to relieve the patients of their depression, irritability and resentment, and place them in an agreeable, quiet and comfortable environment filled with fresh air.

To make the mind relaxed and comfortable in terms of *Qigong* means to "regulate". According to the ancients' sayings, to regulate the heart means "to adjust the disorderly mind and put it into tranquility". It is not mysterious for the mind to enter tranquility. Most people can achieve this.

You feel that the sounds in the surroundings become indistinct. You can hear them, but very indistinctly. You can feel your own breath—both exhaling and inhaling. Sometimes you think of nothing; sometimes your mind is full of distracting thoughts, but you can get rid of them when you are aware of them. A sudden sound may give you a scare. This is preliminary tranquility.

After this you feel half asleep. You are perplexed with your own whereabouts. The sounds around you seem to be far away. You feel your body enlarged or shrunken in size, now heavy, now light. You are even hallucinating in various ways. When your mind concentrates on an object outside the body, you feel as if you were travelling in wonderlands. When you concentrate on a part of your body, you feel the opening and closing of an orifice. This is the tranquility that has gone a step further on the basis of medical *Qigong*.

"In the emptiness, you see an image. The image arouses your emotions. Emotions help you form a more colorful image. From the images you obtain emptiness." This is the state as Laozi said "Obtain emptiness and maintain tranquility". Under this circumstance, a man's mind is, like still water, free from vain hopes. As Li Shizhen said, "When the mind is concentrated upon the inner channels, the performer is able to look within his own self." A person can feel the channels along which his vital energy flows, This is a higher stage of tranquility.

When one's mind is tranquilized after some *Qigong* exercise, not only all disturbances stop, but there is a quiescent and comfortable sensation. This is a feeling produced by the deep inhibitory state of the cerebral cortex—a state of rest for the cerebral cortex. This feeling helps to enhance the patient's confidence to struggle against the disease, to destroy the vicious circle and to enable the cerebral cortex to control the excitement and inhibition of the whole nervous system of the body. When a disease occurs, on the cerebral cortex, there will occur some excited spots of the disease corresponding to different organs and limbs of the body. Thus, a pathological reflex is formed. The cerebral cortex

60

can be inhibited in some special ways by regulating the mind and entering the state of tranquility in the course of *Qigong* training. Fatigue will gradually disappear. Normal function will be restored and diseases will be cured.

Mental *Daoyin* as a *Qigong* technique can be summarized as the following three kinds:

(1) To Concentrate on Inner Objects: This means that the mind is absorbed in concentration of some orifice of your own body, for example, an upper orifice, a lower orifice, a middle orifice, a part of the body, a route of a channel, a solid organ or a hollow organ and so on.

(2) To Concentrate on Outer Objects: This means that the mind is absorbed in concentration of some object outside the body, for example, a rock, a tree or an object.

(3) To Concentrate on Inner-Outer Objects or Non-Inner and Non-Outer Objects: For example, the sounds of exhaling and inhaling; the movements of the body and the figures of silent counting.

In the self-controlled *Qigong* therapy, we consider the last as the main concentration method. This method is easy, safe and effective, free of abstruseness. When he is recovered from his illness, the individual can concentrate his mind either on an inner object or an outer object to further strengthen his health.

Chapter 6

Function of Breathing *Daoyin* (Breath-Regulating Method)

The breathing art in *Qigong* training is breath-regulating. To regulate breath is aimed at breathing in the essential *Qi*. The function of breathing in and out essential *Qi* is to inhale large amounts of oxygen and exhale carbon dioxide through an air exchange in the lungs. So in ancient times *Qigong* was called "Expulsion and Acceptance".

I. Mechanism and Function of Breathing *Daoyin*

In the processes of metabolism, tissue cells incessantly consume oxygen and produce carbon dioxide. Any lack of oxygen will cause pathological changes to the body's organs and their functions. Tissues of the brain are especially easy to be damaged and problems of the function of the central nervous system are caused. On the other hand, if the carbon dioxide is not expelled out of the body in time, respiratory acid poisoning is sure to occur.

In the state of quiescence, the human body inhales about 300 millilitres of oxygen and exhales about 250 millilitres of carbon dioxide through the lung. During strenuous exercise or labour the rate of gaseous interchange can be ten times higher. The vital capacity of an average adult is about 500 millilitres. A skilled practitioner of *Qigong* can have a vital capacity of 5,000—7,000 millilitres. An increase of vital capacity will no doubt benefit the metabolism of the human body. The effectuation of respiratory function is not only dependent on the activities of the respiratory organs and the cooperation with the circulation system, but also is regulated by the spirits and body fluid. Modern medicine holds that the effectuation of respiratory function involves three processes: external respiration, air delivery and internal respiration.

External respiration is a gaseous interchange that takes place in the blood of the capillaries of the pulmonary circulation after the air is taken in through the respiratory tract.

Air delivery is the process of air delivery in the blood between the capillaries of the pulmonary circulation and the general circulation.

Internal respiration is the gaseous interchange between the blood of the capillaries of the general circulation and tissue cells.

From the above-mentioned respiratory processes, it can be seen that blood circulation plays the role of a bridge between the alveoli of the lungs and the various kinds of tissue cells. The respiratory system and the circulation system are closely connected in function. Blood circulation is controlled by the heart, but the blood can reach various parts of the body only when lung-energy flows uninterruptedly. A second function of the lung is to distribute the nutrients to the whole body. This is how the lung acts on postnatal

Qi.

We say the lung controls *Qi*, but does it act on prenatal *Qi* in a way? The lung's function is as follows: water is taken into the stomach and transported upwards through the spleen to the lung; with the descent lung-energy water flows downwards and goes to the kidney; the turbid part of the water is expelled out of the body through the bladder and the clear part will be changed into vital energy at the "triple warmer" and goes up to the lung, where it is circulated and changed into water and descends into the kidney. The circulation goes on and on to maintain the balance of the body's fluid metabolism. The kidney stores the essential *Qi*. The essence of prenatal *Qi* is stored in the kidney. The kidney and the lung are closely related to each other. The essential *Qi* stored in the kidney is supplemented by postnatal *Qi* so as to bring into full play the motive force of the prenatal *Qi*. Modern medical researches have revealed that the lung has the function to produce prostaglandin which is responsible for oestrus.

II. Breath-Regulating, an Inseparable Means to Regulate the Heart

"To count the breath", "to hold the breath", "to observe the breath", "to return to breath", "to purify the breath" and "to follow the breath" are six different ways to regulate the breath in order to tranquilize the mind in varying degrees. According to the tranquility requirements of the self-controlled *Qigong* therapy, "to count the breath" can be adopted, i. e., one exhaling and one inhaling make up one breath.

Aberrations of the mind can be expelled during walking by counting the number of breaths silently. "To follow the breath" means to contemplate the exhaling and inhaling without counting them. The mind follows the breath dependently, free from distracting thoughts. Of course, the method of "listening to the breath" may also be adopted. This method is used to achieve tranquility by listening to the sounds of one's own breathing. It is an extra method of the six breath-regulating methods. Besides, breath-regulating has also the function of arousing true *Qi* so as to regulate blood and vital energy.

Ⅱ. **Breath-Regulating Methods and Their Functions**

The Breath-Regulating and *Qi*-Reenforcing Pattern of *Qigong* exercise has six kinds of breathing *daoyin* methods, i.e., exhaling, inhaling, deep exhaling, breath-holding, blowing and aspirating. Exhaling and inhaling refer to "normal breathing". But the "normal breathing" in *Qigong* differs from the "normal breathing" in daily life. This is a kind of "normal breathing" under the prerequisite of tranquility. Deep breathing refers to deep exhaling through the mouth, which must be followed by corresponding or less deep inhaling. Deep exhaling can excite the parasympathetic nerves so as to dilate the blood vessels, to bring down the blood pressure, to decrease the cholesterol and ease the heartbeats. "To hold the breath" is adopted as a method for the further deepening of breath. "Blowing" refers to the inhaling and exhaling through the nose. This breathing, also called "windy breathing", is a kind of shallow breathing with some slight sounds. As a nasal breathing, this kind of breathing has the function to purify and warm the air that passes through the nasal tract, which is favourable to the lung. Moreover, as a result of the air oscillation, the pituitary gland is stimulated. So the function of the endocrine system is strengthened or regulated. The word *"he"* (aspirating) refers to the pronunciation of certain Chinese characters. The pronouncing method is based on the sounds particularly possessed by the heart, the liver, the spleen, the lung and the kidney as described in *"Nei Jing"*. The choice of the number of times pronounced for each character is based on the same source. Through the echoing of some organs aroused by the oscillation of sounds, pronunciation has the effect to set the involuntary muscles in motion voluntarily by mental control. This has some medical effects.

There are various breathing ways to regulate the breath: abdominal breathing, body breathing, rhythmic breathing and so on. Abdominal breathing is most common. Abdominal breathing is divided into "normal breathing" and "paradoxical breathing". Normal abdominal breathing involves swelling up of the abdomen when inhaling, and contracting the abdomen when exhaling. Paradoxical breathing involves swelling up of the abdomen when exhaling and contracting the abdomen when inhaling. This is a very important breathing method. But when the self-controlled *Qigong* therapy is used to treat diseases, for the sake of alleviating the patients' burden, this method is not encouraged.

Chapter 7
Function of Postural *Daoyin*
(Body-Regulating Method)
and *Daoyin* with Instrument

The posture of *Qigong* training is a kind of pose that the body adopts in the course of exercising. To gain a better effect from *Qigong* exercise, the performer must have his mind tranquilized (to be in the state of tranquility), his "joints relaxed and tendons toned", and his muscles and joints loosened and softened. The purpose of postural *daoyin* is to relax the joints and tone the tendons.

I . Function of *Dao*

"*Dao*" plays a leading role in the self-controlled therapy of *Qigong* training. For *dao* suggests that the cerebral cortex be in the state of protective inhibition, i.e. in the state of tranquility. It is only in this state that the internal energy can flow normally, that the healthy energy within the body can be invigorated and the blood can circulate uninterruptedly. As a result, complaints and ailments will be eliminated. In terms of *Qigong* this is called "the spirit commands vital energy and vital energy commands blood". *Dao* is an important *Qigong* technique with tranquility as its leading factor. *Dao* is "a cardinal remedy" used to cure diseases or to strengthen health.

The self-controlled therapy of *Qigong* exercise takes tranquility as *dao*. Tranquility means that the mental activities are in the state of inhibition. Tranquility dominates all the postures. *"Dao"*, as we understand, means that when the performer practises *Qigong* as a medical therapy, he has his mind tranquilized and inhibited through the whole course of exercise and then he has some better effects. That is why it is called "a cardinal remedy" in treating diseases. But so far this refers to mental activities. Physically *dao* is expressed in "relaxation". Physical relaxation can help the mind get further tranquilized. The following is the key point to achieve both relaxation and tranquility: Relax and tranquilize naturally. Do not intentionally concentrate on only one of the two. Meet the requirements of every *Qigong* pattern in a natural way, i.e. have all the muscles and joints relaxed in a state of tranquility.

I. The Function of **Yin**

"*Yin*" means "to go ahead of the rest". It is like an added ingredient in a decoction of medicine. Though it isn't the main ingredient of the medicine, it helps bring the effect of the medicine into full play. This means "to seek quiescence through motion" and take motion as *yin*." To have both *yin* and *dao* combined means "to take both motion and quiescence into consideration". This is the second key point in the self-controlled therapy of *Qigong* exercise.

About one third of the signals transmitted by the cerebral cortex come from or are sent out by the two hands—especially the palms. So the palms have stronger magnetic fields than other parts of the body. Any change of the position or any movement of the palms can change the direction or position of the magnetic fields of the hands. So the technique to guide the internal energy to flow according to the movements and changes of the magnetic fields of the hands is called "postural *yin*" or "postural *daoyin*". The aim of the postural *daoyin* is to promote the *yang*-energy.

II. Function of Massage (Hand-Massage)

In his *Causes of Diseases*, Zheng Wenzhuo says: "In ancient times massage was a kind of body exercise. ... It can activate all the joints so that the four limbs will be nimble. A person keeps fit through exercise in the same way as a wooden door-hinge avoids being eaten by worms through movements." In his description of massage, he says that hand-massage itself has the function of activating the joints. Wherever hand-massage is applied, the disease is cured as a result of the functions of the hand's infrared radiation, currents of static electricity and particle streams.

The hand connects the six channels of the three-*yang* and three-*yin* (The foot also connects the six channels of the three-*yang* and three-*yin*). Each channel has five kinds of points: the *Jing* (well) points, the *Ying* (brook) points, the *Shu* (transportation) points, the *Jing* (channel) points and the *He* (confluence) points. *Jing* (well) means water source, suggesting abundant vital energy. *Ying* means water in a brook, indicating that channel-energy is still weak. *Shu* means transportation, suggesting vigorous vital energy. *Jing*

69

(channel) means that the vital energy flows vigorously and uninterruptedly. *He* means going into the body, suggesting that the channel energy flows into the body and converges into the solid and hollow organs.

The function of hand-massage is to activate the five points of the hand as well as the wrist joints, the palm joints, and the finger joints so as to strengthen, through *daoyin*, all the joints of the whole body in cooperation with the toe-raised foot. This is the significance of relaxing the joints and toning the tendons.

To apply the vital energy of the hand and bring it back to benefit one's own body, it is necessary to reenforce mental *daoyin*, i.e., "to unite mental activities and vital energy as one". This is the third key point of the self-controlled *Qigong* therapy. The Head-Massage Tranquilizing Pattern is an example in utilizing this massage technique. Its mechanism and function are as follows:

The head, where the cerebrum and other higher nerves of the body are located, is the centre that controls the whole body. Traditional Chinese medicine calls it "the headquarters of all *yang*-channels". Head-Massage Tranquilizing Pattern of *Qigong* training is designed to relieve anxiety and regulate *yang* by massaging the various points on the head, so as to rectify the general unbalanced state of *yin* and *yang*. The Head-Massage Tranquilizing Pattern, a major *Qigong* technique to treat coronary diseases, has the function to relieve anxiety and calm the heart. It can eliminate the excitement of the cerebral cortex, help the cerebrum get relaxed and tranquilized, regulate the nerve centre of the blood vessels, and promote the blood vessels to dilate and contract regularly. Head-massage has a very good effect in treating both cerebral angiosclerosis and coronary sclerosis. The following is a table of its indications.

Table 3 Channels and Points of the "Head-Massaging" and Diseases to Be Treated

Massage sequence	Point No.	Name of point	Name of Channel	Indications	Functions
1	1	Yintang	Extra-ordinary Points	frontal headache dizziness, eye trouble, nose trouble, hyper-tension	to link up the Du Channel and the Ren Channel
	2	Baihui	The Du Channel	headache, dizzi-ness and hypertension	
	3	Shuaigu	The Gall-bladder Channel	cephalalgia, lateral headache, depression, vomiting	to dredge the chan-nels
	4	Fengfu	The Du Channel	cold, headache, stiff neck, apoplexy	
2	5	Yangbai	The Gall-bladder Channel	frontal headache, sore eye, insomnia, facial paralysis,	to recuperate the depleted yang and relieve mental uneasiness
	6	Tianzhu	The Urinary Bladder Channel	occipital heada-che, stiff neck, neurasthenia	

Massage sequence	Point No.	Name of point	Name of Channel	Indications	Functions
3	7	Touwei	The Stomach Channel	migraine, dizziness, eye trouble	to stop the wind-evil and invigorate the brain
	8	Fengchi	The Gallbladder Channel	apoplexy, hemiplegia, ear trouble, cold, headache, eye trouble, rhinitis	
4	9	Taiyang	Extraordinary Points	eye trouble, headache	to expel heat and improve eyesight
	10	Sizhu-kong	The Sanjiao Channel	migraine, eye trouble, facial paralysis	
5	11	Tinghui	The Small Intestine Channel	ear trouble and fullness of abdomen	to regulate the vital energy and blood
	12	Xiaguan	The Stomach Channel	ear trouble, toothache, facial paralysis	
6	13	Qing-ming	The Urinary Bladder Channel	conjuntivitis and other eye trouble	
7	14	Ying-xiang	The Large Intestine Channel	rhinitis, stuffy nose, excessive nasal discharge, rapid respiration, edema	
	15	Cheng-jiang	The Ren Channel	diabetes, lockjaw	

IV. Function of Toe-Raised Step

Toe-raised step is an exercise of the foot joints. It can treat the diseases of the five solid organs. Besides it can arouse the internal energy of the spleen and the liver, and promote the internal energy of the body to rise and flow vigorously and uninterruptedly so as to reenforce the function of the vital energy and blood. Touching the heel to the ground with the toes raised can activate the *Qiao*-Channels of *yin* and *yang* (These two channels originate from the centre of the heel) so that the internal energy coming out from the *yin*-channel can go in through the *yang*-channel and the internal energy coming out from the *yang*-channel can go in through the *yin*-channel. So the channels are dredged and *yin* and *yang* regulated.

Generally speaking, the internal energy of the body varies with age and health conditions. As his case is getting worse, the patient will have asthenia-syndrome in the lower part and sthenia in the upper part of his body. This is caused by the insufficiency of the energy in the liver and kidney channels. Symptoms of the asthenia-syndrome of the lower part include lumbago and pain in the knee, fatigue and emission. Symptoms of the sthenia-syndrome of the upper part include dizziness, conjunctivitis, hypochondriac pain and irritation. To improve this condition, the self-controlled *Qi-gong* therapy is designed to stimulate the tiptoe with the toe-raised posture, so as to invigorate the energy of the liver and spleen channels. On the other hand, the heel is also stimulated so as to promote the flowing of the bladder and kidney-energy (as in the case of the Breath-Regulating and *Qi*-Reenforcing Pattern).At the same time when moving his foot, the performer should concentrate his mind on the lower part of his body so as to guide the abnormal rising of lung-energy to go downward. This will relieve the sthenia-syndrome of the upper part. The coordination between the upper part and lower part is aimed at regulating the sthenia of the upper part.

V. Function of the Relaxed and Quiescent Qi-Regulating Pattern (With a Stick)

The technique of this *Qigong* pattern is to knead the *Laogong* Point, which is at the centre of the palm with a wooden stick. The *Laogong* Point belongs to the Channel of the Pericardium—the protective envelope of the heart. The purpose of this exercise is to make the heart and the liver coordinate in function and play a better role in blood circulation. The liver stores blood while the heart controls blood circulation. So the insufficiency of heart-blood can lead to deficiency of liver-blood, and on the other hand, the insufficiency of liver-blood can lead to the deficiency of heart-blood. To reenforce the Channels of the Pericardium is to reenforce the function of the heart so as to invigorate blood circulation and nourish the liver. Besides, the liver serves to regulate the activity of vital energy, while the heart controls mental and emotional activities. Any mental disorder caused by liver trouble often affects the heart, and on the other hand, mental disorder due to heart trouble also affects the liver. For example, the insufficiency of liver-blood leads to dizziness (most likely insomnia, palpitation with fear and so on); the insufficiency of heart-*yang* often leads to the flaring up of asthenic fire (symptoms of liver trouble such as impetuosity, irritation, dizziness, insomnia and conjunctivitis). So kneading the *Laogong* Point not only treats the heart, it also treats the liver. This method, as traditional Chinese medicine calls it, is "a treatment aimed at the root cause of the disease".

In the Relaxed and Quiescent Qi-Regulating Pattern, the waist exercise plays a leading role. For example, dropping, bending, relaxing and turning of the waist all belong to the activities that invigorate the circulation of the kidney-energy, in addition to their function of regulating the liver channel. The liver stores blood while the kidney stores the essence of life. Physiologically, only when the kidney-essence nourishes the liver, can the liver function normally. However, an abundant store of kidney-essence depends on the sufficient supply of the liver-blood. Pathologically, the insufficiency of liver-blood can lead to asthenia of the kidney-essence; the insufficiency of kidney-essence can lead to the insufficiency of the liver-blood, and therefore, the asthenia-syndrome of both the liver and the kidney occurs. The insufficiency of the kidney-*yin* can lead to the insufficiency of the liver-*yin* and the sthenia-syndrome of the liver-*yang*. To reenforce the function of the kidney, the liver must be first nourished. This is called "water nourishes wood".

"The liver serves to regulate the activity of vital energy". This means that the liver-energy has the physiological function of smoothing, lifting, nourishing and regulating the

75

vital energy. Only when the liver-energy is smoothed and regulated, can the vital energy and blood flow freely and the performer will feel comfortable and at ease. If there is any pathological change in the liver, the liver's regulating and smoothing function will be disturbed. So the liver-energy will become stagnated with symptoms such as tightness in the chest, hypochondriac pain, depression, abnormal menstruation and so on. Sthenia of the liver-energy often leads to impetuosity, irritation, insomnia and dreaminess, dizziness and so on. The Relaxed and Quiescent Qi-regulating Pattern is desinged to utilize the specific function of the liver: The liver stores blood while the heart circulates it. When a person is moving, the blood flows in all the channels. When a person is in the state of quiescence, the blood returns to the liver." The Relaxed and Quiescent Qi-regulating Pattern emphasizes the flow and circulation of vital energy and blood, so as to bring into full play the liver's function of regulating and smoothing the activities of the vital energy. When a person is relaxed and quiescent, the blood returns to the liver and nourishes it, and the liver will give full play to its function of storing blood. So the Relaxed and Quiescent Qi-regulating Pattern is desinged in consideration of the liver's function as well as its reception of nourishment.

Chapter 8
Application of the Technique of Self-Controlled *Qigong* Therapy

I. **Time for *Qigong* Exercise**

The changes of the natural atmosphere affect the changes inside the human body. The internal energy flows inside the human body according to its own law along the Twelve Channels. The Twelve Channels are connected end to end, forming a circulation passage.

The traditional Chinese medicine holds that in a day's time "the internal energy flows in the Gallbladder Channel during the period from 23 o'clock to 1 o'clock ...; the internal energy flows in the Heart Channel during the period from 11 to 13." It takes one day for the earth to make one rotation just as it takes one day for the internal energy to make one circle in flowing. So there is a regularity of the flowing time corresponding to the Twelve Channels. The regularity is as follows:

The period of time	The channel in which the internal energy flows
23 to 1	The Gallbladder Channel
1 to 3	The Liver Channel
3 to 5	The Lung Channel

5 to 7	The Large Intestine Channel
7 to 9	The Stomach Channel
9 to 11	The Spleen Channel
11 to 13	The Heart Channel
13 to 15	The Small Intestine Channel
15 to 17	The Urinary Bladder Channel
17 to 19	The Kidney Channel
19 to 21	The Pericardium Channel
21 to 23	The *Sanjiao* Channel

The channel in which the internal energy flows most vigorously during the specific period contains the most exuberant internal energy. For example, The Breath-Regulating and *Qi*-Reenforcing Pattern, which is a kind of lung-channel *Qigong* pattern, should be performed from 3:00 to 5:00. As The Large Intestine Channel and The Lung Channel share a paired relationship, it is also advisable to perform the lung-channel *Qigong* pattern from 5:00 to 7:00. From 3:00 to 7:00, the internal energy flows in the Lung Channel and The Large Intestine Channel. The lung is responsible for astringency, During this period, the energy of the rising sun is responsible for birth. "Birth and astringency" are like a hungry baby sucking the breast to his heart's content. So it is most effective to perform the Breath-Regulating and *Qi*-Reenforcing Pattern during this period. As for seasons, the atmosphere in spring and summer belongs to *yang*, so breath should be regulated with *yin*. The atmosphere in autumn and winter belongs to *yin*, so breath should be regulated with *yang*. From 3:00 to 5:00, the internal energy passes through the lung, which is one of the five viscera and belongs to *yin*, so this period is most suitable for *Qigong* practice. The internal energy passes through the large intestine from 5:00 to 7:00 and the large intestine is among the six hollow organs and belongs to *yang*, so this period is quite good for practising *Qigong* in autumn.

Because The Head-Massaging and Mind-Tranquilizing Pattern is aimed at strengthening the Heart Channel, it is best to perform this pattern during the period from eleven to thirteen, but it can also be performed during the period from nineteen to twenty-one. The Kidney-Massaging and Essence-Benefiting Pattern is designed to strengthen the kidney. So it is best to perform this pattern during the period from 17:00 to 19:00. If this period is inconvenient, it is also possible to perform it during the period from 15:00 to 17:00 when the internal energy passes through the Urinary Bladder Channel. It is also good to perform it during the period from 21:00 to 23:00 when the internal energy flows in the *Sanjao* Channel.

The Toe-Raised Transport and Conversion Pattern is aimed at soothing the spleen and the stomach. The spleen is amidst the internal organs, so this pattern can be performed at any time except when the scorching sun is directly overhead so as to prevent the internal energy from rising rapidly, which may lead to overabundance of *yang*. It is appropriate to perform the *Qigong* patterns related with the Spleen Channel and Stomach Channel in the period from 7:00 to 11:00.

The Relaxed and Quiescent *Qi*-Regulating Pattern is a

method to strengthen the liver. The liver-energy flows most smoothly during the period from 1:00 to 3:00, but it is quite inconvenient to practise *Qigong* during the small hours. So, in order to promote the vigorous flow of the vital energy and blood, this pattern can be performed in the after-noon, which can benefit the health to some extent.

II. Directions for *Qigong* Exercise

A good site for *Qigong* exercise is in a forest (especially in pine and cypress woods). With a hill at the back and water on the sides, the air is particularly fresh. The direction of per-formance is of secondary importance. However, as the sun rises in the east, the energy from the east, which is called *Shaoyang*, has the same quality as the liver-energy; when the sun turns to the south, the energy from the south, which is called *Laoyang*, has the same quality as the heart-energy; when the sun sets in the west, the energy from the west, which is called *Shaoyin*, has the same quality as the lung-energy; when the sun disap-pears in the north, the energy from the morth, which is called *Laoyin*, has the same quality as the spleen-energy. Under the influence of similar *Qi*s seeking each other, the chest and abdomen are connected with the earthly *Qi* as *yin*, while the back is connected with the heavenly *Qi* as *yang*. The direction of the back, which is connected with heavenly *Qi*, means tonifying and the direction of the chest and abdomen means purging. Most people who suffer from chronic diseases have overabundance of *yang* in the upper part and deficiency of the primordial energy in the lower part. So they should face the south for most of the time. When facing the south, the chest and abdomen can pull the heart-energy downward and the back reenforces the kidney-energy.

II. Diseases Treated with Various *Qigong* Patterns

The five fundamental *Qigong* patterns are desinged to strengthen the vital energy circulating in the channels of the five solid organs respectively. There are eight extra-channels besides the Twelve Channels. The Eight Extra-Channels are not directly connected with the viscera, but they are special passages to regulate the five solid organs and six hollow organs through the Twelve Channels.

The Head-Massaging and Mind-Tranquilizing Pattern can treat diseases related with the Heart Channel, the Small Intestine Channel, the Pericardium Channel and the *Du* Channel; the Relaxed and Quiescent *Qi*-Regulating Pattern can treat diseases related with the Liver Channel, the Pericardium Channel, the Heart Channel, the Gallbladder Channel and the Kidney Channel; the Toe-Raised Transport and Conversion Pattern can treat diseases related with the Spleen Channel, the Stomach Channel, the Heart Channel, the *Dai* Channel, the *Ren* Channel, the *Chong* Channel, the *Yinqiao* Channel, the *Yangqiao* Channel and the *Yinwei* Channel; the Breath-Regulating and *Qi*-Reenforcing Pattern can treat diseases related with the Lung Channel, the Large Intestine Channel, the *Ren* Channel, the *Chong* Channel, the *Yinqiao* Channel, the *Yangqiao* Channel and the *Yangwei* Channel; the Kidney-Massaging and Essence-Benefiting Pattern can treat diseases related with the Kidney Channel and the Urinary Bladder Channel. The following is a table showing the diseases treated by various patterns.

Table 4   Diseases Treated by Various
                Qigong Patterns

Qigong Patterns	Viscera	Functions	Indications
1. Head-Massaging and Mind-Tranquilizing Pattern (to be accompanied by Kidney-Massaging and Essence-Benefiting Pattern)	heart	to control blood circulation	deficiency of heart-energy, weak pulse, stagnation of blood circulation, proiosystole, cyanotic lips
2. Breath-Regulating and Qi-Reenforcing Pattern (the Heart-Strengthening Method)	pericardium	to control emotions	fidget, insomnia, dreaminess, restlessness, delirium, amnesia
		to control perspiration	excessive sweating, nervousness and palpitation caused by the consumption of body fluid
		the tongue being the orifice to the pericardium	red tongue, erosion of the tongue, curled-up tongue, stiff tongue, purplish tongue,
		to protect the heart	loss or partial loss of consciousness, delirious speech
3. Relaxed and Quiescent Qi-Regulating Pattern (to be accompanied by the Blowing Methods to strengthen the kidney,	liver	to store blood, to smooth and regulate the flow of vital energy	blood stasis due to stagnation of Qi, irregular menstruation, amenorrhoea, flushed face and red eye, vomiting blood, metrorrhagia, irritability, insomnia and dreaminess, dizziness, thoracic tightness and abdominal distension, hypochondriac distension and pain

Qigong Patterns	Viscera	Functions	Indications
the liver, the spleen and the lung and "Aspirating" method for amenorrhea	liver	to determine the condition of the tendons	stiffness or spasm of tendons, tremor of hands and feet, numbness in the body and limbs, difficult flexion
		the eye being the orifice to the liver	dryness and uneasy feeling of the eye, night blindness, conjunctivitis, swollen and sore eyes, pterygium
4. Toe-Raised Transport and Conversion Pattern	spleen	to transport, distribute, and transform nutrients and promote water metabolism	abdominal distension, diarrhea, malnutrition, phlegm due to accumulation of water, edema
		to govern blood	bloody stool, metrorrhagia
		to nourish the muscles and the limbs	muscular flaccidity and atrophy, general weakness and fatigue
		the mouth being the orifice to the spleen	dyspepsia, pale lips
5. Breath-Regulating and Qi-	Lung	to control vital energy and govern respiration	shortness of breath and general weakness, aphasia, general fatigue

Qigong Patterns	Viscera	Functions	Indications
Reeforcing Pattern	Lung	to activate the flow of vital energy, blood and body fluid and, lung-energy keeping pure and descendant	fullness in the chest, stuffy nose, productive cough, tightness in the chest, rapid respiration (trachitis and bronchitis
		to control skin and hair, the nose being the orifice to the lung	pale skin and dry hair, haggard face, abnormal sweating rhinitis, sinusitis, laryngitis, pharyngitis
6. Kidney-Massage and Essence-Benefiting Pattern	Kidney	to store essence of life and to be responsible for growth and reproduction	hypogonadism, senility, premature senility
		to aid the lung in regulating respiration	rapid respiration
		to control the bone and nourish the bone marrow connected with the brain	fragile bone, shaky teeth, hypomnesia, listlessness
		the ear being the orifice to the kidney, to govern urination and defecation	tinnitus, hypoacusis incontinence of urine and stool

Chapter 9
Epilogue—*Qigong* and the Control of One's Life

I. Control of the Internal Pathogenic Factors

As the saying goes: "A disease is cured more by recuperation than by medication." This means recuperation is far more important than medical treatment. The *Qigong* therapy will be more effective if the day is divided as 8 hours for sleep, 4 hours for *Qigong* practice, 12 hours for work and rest, and the performer's work and life are in accordance with the flowing law of the internal energy. If the performer's work and life run counter to the flowing law of the internal energy, not only the effect of *Qigong* therapy will be counteracted, but also the disease will be aggravated. From this we can see clearly that it is very important for the *Qigong* practitioner to make a good arrangement of his daily work and life.

In their daily life activities, people are often involved in the seven modes of emotions—joy, anger, grief, over-thinking, sadness, terror and fright. All this is closely related with the viscera. The traditional Chinese medicine holds that the disorder of liver may cause anger. The heart controls joy. The disorder of spleen may cause grief and over-thinking.

The disorder of the lung may cause sadness. The kidney is easily affected by fright. Under normal circumstances, the seven modes of emotional activities are good to health. For example, appropriate anger helps disperse the depressed liver-energy. So it has the function to prevent stasis of liver-energy. However, rage should be avoided. For rage may lead to the abnormal rising of the internal energy, which may result in flushed face and ears, dyspnea and shortness of breath. Violent and uncontrolled anger may lead to disorder of the liver, injury of the eye, syncope, cerebral hemorrhage or even death. It is the same case with joy. Under normal circumstances, joy makes a person feel comfortable because his heart-energy flows smoothly. So joy has the function to disperse the depressed heart-energy. Yet excessive joy may lead to the sluggishness of vital energy. Consequently, the heart-energy lacks activity, unable to go upward to nourish the mind, and therefore functional disorder of the brain and heart will occur. Severe cases may be fatal. Any fluctuation of the seven modes of emotions will lead to unnecessary consumption or damage of internal energy. So the vital energies flowing along the channels of viscera will be out of harmony, which causes abnormal activity of the vital energy and functional disorder of the cerebral cortex. These are internal pathogenic factors. *Qigong* practitioners and patients who practise *Qigong* for the treatment of diseases, must avoid any fluctuation of emotions. Otherwise they will not only aggravate their cases but also lose all the achievements they have made through their long-term *Qigong* exercise.

To prevent the fluctuation of emtions, a *Qigong* performer must do more good deeds, so that the heart is light and the mind is completely at ease. When involved in sudden agitation, you should concentrate your mind on the downward pulling force and relax the body and the four limbs so as to effectively avoid any large consumption or disorder of the internal energy. When you feel that your emotions or the emotions of another person are likely to fluctuate, you may try to regulate and control your emotions with emotions so that the visceral energy which is going to explode is restrained and calmed down.

The relationship between a person's emotions and his viscera was one of the beliefs of the theory of the five elements in ancient China. This theory can be applied not only to the human body, but also to the nature. This is shown in the following table:

Table 5

	Nature				
five flavors	five colors	five conversions	five atmospheric influences	five directions	five seasons
sour	blue	birth	wind	east	spring
bitter	red	growth	summer heat	south	summer
sweet	yellow	conversion	wetness	centre	long summer
acrid	white	astringent	dryness	west	autumn
salty	black	storage	cold	north	winter

five elements	Human Body				
	five solid organs	six hollow organs	five sense organs	physical appearance	emotions
wood	liver	gallbladder	the eye	tendon	anger
fire	heart	triple warmer & small intestine	the tongue	pulse	joy
earth	spleen	stomach	the mouth	muscle	over-thinking
metal	lung	large intestine	the nose	skin & hair	sorrow
water	kidney	urinary bladder	the ear	bone	terror

The five elements have an interpromoting and interacting (checking) relationship. "To interpromote" means to foster and encourage birth and growth. "To interact" means to restrain and restrict.

The sequence of the interpromoting relationship of the five elements is: wood generates fire; fire generates earth; earth generates metal; metal generates water; water generates wood. This circle is endless. The sequence of the interacting (conquering) relationship of the five elements is: wood restricts earth; earth restricts water; water restricts fire; fire restricts metal; metal restricts wood. This restricting circle is also endless. This restricting relationship can be applied to the problems of emotions. For example, anger belongs to the rising of exuberant liver-energy which can be counteracted by the descending lung-energy. The lung controls sadness and sadness may lead to the consumption of the abnormal rising of liver-energy. Joy belongs to the rapid rising heart-energy. It can be regulated by fright and terror that are controlled by the rapid descending kidney-energy. Terror may lead to the abnormal falling of vital energy, so it can pull downward the abnormal rapid rising of heart-energy. Excessive sadness may lead to the extravagant consumption of the lung-energy, which damages *yin* and the heart. Consumption of the lung-energy can be remitted by heart-energy of joy. Excessive terror may lead to the abnormal falling of vital energy. Fright may lead to the dispersion of vital energy. Excessive fright and terror may lead to the abnormal sinking of essential energy, which damages kidney-energy. Over-thinking can be applied for mental control. Over-thinking can lead vital energy in assembling, so it helps bring back the dispersed energy. Overthinking and anxiety may lead to the depression and stagnation of vital energy, which results in weak transporting and converting ability of the spleen-energy and lack of appetite. Mild cases have dyspepsia, abdominal distention and diarrhea. In severe cases, the blood and vital energy will be stagnated in the chest and abdomen, causing a feeling of fullness in the chest or the upper abdomen. This stagnated ever-sinking spleen-energy can be smoothed and aroused by stimulating, with a feeling of anger, the liver-energy that goes upward and outward. In short, hyperactivity of *yin* is treated with *yang* so as to check the unnecessary consumption of internal energy and promote a mild *yin*-energy with *yang*-energy hidden. So the blood and vital energy can flow uninterruptedly and diseases can be prevented.

II. Control of Exogenous Pathogenic Factors

The external pathogenic factors are the six evil-factors that are related to the human body, i.e., wind, fire, heat, wetness, dryness and cold. These six evil-factors exist outside the body. Each of them has a bias. They, like the seven modes of emotions, are good for the human body under normal circumstances. But they can be harmful to the body when some abnormal phenomena occur. For example, if it is not cold in winter and not hot in summer, which is called unseaonable weather, the weather can easily make people sick. If the weather is too cold or too hot for the human body to tolerate, the normal flowing of the internal energy will be disturbed and diseases will occur. *Qigong* practitioners should protect themselves from being attacked by the six evil-factors.

III. Control of Miscellaneous Factors

Be Moderate in Eating and Drinking. If the food is too cold, the cold-evil will render the vital energy sluggish, so the channels and collaterals will be blocked. Blockage will cause pain and damage to the stomach and intestines. The small intestine is connected with the heart and the large intestine is connected with the lung. So extremely cold food will not only damage the stomach and intestines, but also affect the heart and lung. Extremely hot food will let out internal energy and damage the blood and vital energy. Excessive heat, especially smoking and alcohol, may bring on cold. The cold-evil renders the vital energy sluggish and causes stasis of blood and vital energy. Excessive eating may cause sthenia and upward perverse of stomach-energy, which damages the spleen and stomach. Too greasy food may damage the stomach-energy and causes serious cases of furuncle and pyogenic infections and ulcerous diseases of skin. So one should not eat extremely cold, hot, or too greasy food or eat to excess.

Give No Partiality to Particular Kinds of Food. If the food is limited to only a few flavours, the internal energy will be damaged. For example, as the lung controls vital energy, it is very powerful in absorbing acrid flavours. Acrid food can be easily absorbed by the lung channel. The lung-energy will spread with the spreading of acrid flavours. An appropriate amount of acrid food may help activate the lung-energy and promote the lung's function. Any excessive intake of acrid food will lead to the great loss or damage of lung-energy. This will be harmful to diseases due to disorder of vital energy. So patients with such diseases should not eat much spicy hot food. Patients with other visceral diseases have similar problems: The salty flavour is likely to spread with blood, and therefore causes blood co-agulation. So patients with heart-trouble should not eat much salty food. The bitter flavour is likely to spread along the bones. Much intake of bitter flavour will lead to hyperactivity of heart-fire and consumption of kidney-fluid. As the kidney controls the bones, patients with diseases of the kidney or bones should not eat much bitter food. The sweet flavour is likely to spread through the muscles. So patients with diseases of the spleen, stomach or muscles should not eat much sweet food. The sour flavour is likely to spread along the tendons and to astringe. Much intake of sour flavour will lead to stiffness of the tendons. So patients with tendon trouble should not eat too much sour food. As the liver controls the tendons, patients with liver trouble should also eat less sour food. Patients who practise *Qigong* as a therapy should give no partiality to particular kinds of food and, especially, should eat less onion, garlic, pepper and so on so as to avoid consumption of internal energy and secure the effect.

Allocate Work and Rest Evenly. "The shape is formed by vital energy". All of the various kinds of shapes of the body are maintained with the support of the internal energy. Any kind of shape or action of the body, if kept unchanged for a long time, will lead to the excessive consumption of the internal energy that supports and maintains it. And the viscera concerned will be injured. The strain of the eye damages blood; lying too much damages vital energy; to remain in the sitting position for a long time damages muscles; standing too long damages the bones; to keep walking for a long time damages the tendons. Walking, standing and looking belong to "work" while sitting and lying belong to "rest" (leisure). Both overwork and inappropriate rest can cause diseases of the viscera as a result of the extravagant consumption of internal energy. So work and rest must alternate. As too much lying damages vital energy, the overuse of the eye damages blood, and blood is "the mother" of vital energy, the damage of blood will lead to the damage of vital energy. So patients who practise *Qigong* should try to avoid lying in bed for long. Besides, excessive sexual intercourse should be avoided. Sexual intercourse consumes the essence of life. Consumption of essence of life damages the kidney and empties the bones of their marrow, and the brain is weakened. So only when the essence of life is abundant can there be exuberant vital energy. Only when there is exuberant vital energy can the *Qigong* therapy be effective. Therefore, during the *Qigong* training period of time, sexual intercourse is preferably suspended. It should also be restrained even when not practising *Qigong*.

Lead a Regular Life. To live in houses and wear clothes are active measures for man to protect himself from being violently attacked by the six factors—wind, fire, summer heat, wetness, dryness and cold. If the wind intrudes the human body violently, the man will suffer from "affection caused by exogenous pathogenic factors". This affection is an antecedent of diseases. The wind exists all the year round. So one must be sure to change clothes in time and be careful not to sleep or lie near a window or wall that is not airtight, so as to avoid being exposed directly to the wind. Other evil factors can also cause problems. The cold-evil is characteristic of astringency. It can block the channels and collaterals, which causes pain and damage of the heart. Summer heat and fire spread excessively. They consume and impair the primordial energy, impair body fluid and the

93

lung. Wetness too easily obstructs the mechanism of vital energy and causes impairment of *yang* Especially in the case of extremely turbid grease stagnation, a person is subjected to be sick and recovers with difficulty. Dryness causes dry skin, throat pain, cough or asthma. So one must be well prepared against the six evil factors. A patient who practises *Qigong* as a therapy should live in a house that suits him for *Qigong* training and wear clothes that fit the smooth flow of the internal energy. For example, tight-fitting clothes and high-heeled shoes will greatly affect the flow of the internal energy. And too heavy or too light clothes can also be unfavourable to the circulation of blood and vital energy, and can interfere with relaxation and tranquility.

Chapter 10
An Approach to the Mechanism of *Qigong* Therapy for Tumours (Cancers)

The tumour, which is a kind of commonly and frequently encountered disease, is often seen with people of 30—50 years of age. And the malignant tumour—cancer, severely threatens the people's health. Therefore, prevention and cure of tumours and cancers by *Qigong* therapy is of great significance in protecting the people's health.

The malignant tumour (cancer) is a disease that is difficult to control in the present world. People in China came to know this disease a long time ago. There were records of tumours in the inscriptions on bones or tortoise shells of the Yin Dynasty ruins. And there were also accounts of "painful swelling of the body surface" in the 12th century B.C. There were detailed accounts of and treatments to tumours in "Nei Jing", the earliest book on medicine available in China. In the chapter "On Uncommon Diseases, Familiar Conversation", it says: " 'mass' should be treated by medicine in combination with daoyin. It cannot be cured with medicine alone." What kind of disease is 'mass'? In another chapter entitled "Origins of Disease, The Spiritual Pivot", it says, "Retention causes mass". Retention has the meaning of "stagnation". It originates from flowing substances within the body such as vital energy and blood. It stagnates because it is attacked by evil factors and gradually takes the form of a lump as a result of its excessive accumulation. The lump is called something like a mass that may subside spontaneously in the traditional Chinese medicine, and nowadays it is called a benign tumour. As for the malignant tumour (It is also called carcinoma, cancer and indurated mass), it is caused mainly by the stagnation and retention of vital energy, blood, phlegm and food.

Through its researches on cancer cells, modern science holds that "a silkworm-cocoon-like protective membrane may be formed around the tumour cell." And this membrane makes it impossible for the giant phagocyte, which is powerful enough to kill the pathogenic bacteria, to approach the cancer cell. Moreover, drugs, or even some powerful radiation can not penetrate the membrane. That is why they say that "cancer can't be cured by drugs alone." To treat cancers, drugs must be combined with *daoyin*.

How can cancer be cured by *Qigong*? To answer this question, we must start with the characteristics of cancer. Neither the body of cancer nor cancer cells are components of the mother body. They are the infant bodies which absorb nourishment and energy from the mother body for their own growth. And they are thus called "the embryos". In accordance with this physiological and pathological mechanism, we adopt "The Blowing and Fast Walking Method" to cure cancer by walking fast and changing the normal breathing so as to destroy the infant "embryos" in the mother body. In this way the cancer cells and carcinoma bodies can be destroyed.

Secondly we use "The Open-and-Close Deep-Breathing Method", "The Aspirating and Word-Pronouncing Method" to treat cancers by changing the normal breathing. For by changing the normal breathing into "rapid blowing", "slow deep-exhaling" or "relaxed aspirating", the blood clots or tumours stagnated or retained in the channels of the body can be dissolved.

How can the changes of normal breathing and fast walking dissolve blood clots and tumours? The reason is as follows: Due to *Qigong*'s function of "regulating the mind", "regulating the breath" and "regulating the physical body" (i.e., tranquility, various kinds of breathing methods and fast walking methods and so on), the internal energy can flow vigorously so that the Ren Channel is smoothed and the Lung Channel is strengthened. In the course of treating "mass", true *Qi is* fostered and the immunity of the body strengthend. It is reported abroad that "persistent physical training activities, which are vigorous enough to make a person's heartbeat increase to 70—80% of his maximum beat rate, can help him to dissolve his blood clots. Other reports believe that "long-distance running can cure cancers". These reports can serve as preliminary interpretations for the *Qigong* principles on the prevention and cure of cancers.

The following is an analysis of the causes of cancer.

Traditional Chinese medicine holds that tumour is a kind of disease involving the whole body. The causes of tumour can be summarized as this: Disorder of internal organs caused by emotional strains and imbalance of viscera let the pathogenic evils enter the body and obstruct the channels and collaterals. The pathogenic evils cause problems and finally the stagnation of blood and vital energy develop into tumours. The development involves a decline of vital energy and a growth of evil factors. The pathology of cancer is as follows:

Stasis of Energy: Emotional strains, depression of liver-energy or external evil factors lead to the stagnation of vital energy. Long-term stagnation of the vital energy will surely cause the stagnation of blood. And the stagnation of blood will gradually cause clots, just as it is said in *"Nei Jing"*:

97

"Inappropriate joy and anger ... cold and heat at the wrong time and the prevailing evil factors will inevitably cause blood clots".

Blood Stasis: The obstruction of vital energy leads to the impedance of the circulation of the blood. The impedance of blood circulation gradully leads to blood stasis. So blood stasis is always complicated by stasis of vital energy. Blood stasis is also called "dead blood". The "dead blood" is retained in a certain place, unable to move about, and eventually develops into a mass.

Retention of Wetness-evil: Debility of the spleen and stomach, and indigestion cause retention of fluid in the body. Long-term retention of fluid will produce toxic materials.

Retention of Phlegm: Functional disorder of the spleen and the lung lead to ill dissolution of the watery food and ill distribution of body fluid. And the retention of water and body fluid will cause phlegm, especially when it is complicated by evil heat. The phlegm is unable to go up. The stagnation of phlegm in the lung leads to asthma, and the stagnation of phlegm in the stomach causes gastric disorder and nausea. When the phlegm goes beneath the skin, it will take the form of a lump.

Toxin Attack: The poisonous evils may come from the external environment or may be generated by the stagnation of heat within the body.

Asthenia of Healthy Energy: Deficiency of both energy and blood, and debility of vital energy make the body vulnerable to attacks by "tumour evils". When "the evils of

98

tumour" intrude the human body, they will damage the blood and energy and make them more and more debilitated. If the vital energy can not be restored, the disease will lead to a vicious circle.

The pathological changes mentioned above may occur either alone or overlappingly, e.g. stasis of vital energy and the stagnation of blood, the coagulation of phlegm and the retention of wetness-evils, mutual affection of phlegm-retention and blood stasis, sthenia of the pathogenic evils and asthenia of the healthy energy. So the choice of Qigong therapy should be based on differentiation of symptoms and signs. Because cancers are caused mainly by emotional strains and by the sthenia of evil factors and asthenia of the healthy energy, stress should be put on reenforcing vital energy and reducing the sthenia of evil factors in the choice of Qigong patterns. To reenforce the primordial energy, the Breath-Regulating and Qi-Reenforcing Pattern is preferably applied, "Fast-Walking Blowing Method" is advisably used to purge sthenia and expel evils. As for the disturbances caused by emotional factors, the Open-and-Close Deep-Exhaling Method" should be applied to tranquilize the mind and keep the cerebral cortex inhibited protectively. To bring into full play the function of Qigong exercises in treating cancers, patients should perform no less than 4 hours (including the breaks) and even 6 hours each time. The patient can take a break after performing for half an hour so as to avoid possible fatigue. More practice will help regain the healthy energy and the patient will feel strong again. More practice will help expel evil factors and inhibit the disease, and reduce the consumption of physical strength. The rapid growth of healthy energy and the fast expulsion of evil factors may lead to earlier restoration of the normal functions of the body and vigorous metabolic activities. So more nourishment is absorbed, delivered and distributed throughout the body, leaving no room for tumour cells to take in. This is a circle of favourable character. However, beginners should not perform for long each time. Performing time can be extended gradually with the increase of the physical strength.

Du Fu, an ancient Chinese poet, says in one of his poems (*March Across the Frontier*): "How I long for the relief of my sorrow, yet the aberrations have been in my mind too long." Only when the mind is free from aberrations, can a person control his mind over sorrow. So "to regulate the mind" is the main *Qigong* technique for a person to relieve himself from the abyss of sorrow. That is to say a person should let optimism prevail over pessimism. In order to foster optimism the individual should practise *Qigong* in addition to other subjective efforts. The practice of *Qigong* not only cultivates vital energy and builds up the performer's health, but also promotes the development of optimism and have a quiescent mind, so as to keep the cerebral cortex in a state of neither excitement nor overinhibition—a state of tranquility. This means an "attack" to cancers. The reason is that tranquility will promote a better circulation of both blood and vital energy, build up the health and strengthen the immunity, so the inhibited cancer cells will gradually perish. Therefore, when practising, patients with cancers must have confidence in conquering the disease, perseverence in doing *Qigong* exercise, and patience in overcoming difficulties.

Book II

THE TECHNIQUE OF
QIGONG

Chapter 1
Starting and Ending Forms of
Basic *Qigong* Exercise Patterns

I. Starting Form

1. The Relaxed and Quiescent Form in Standing Position

   Pithy Formula

   Keep the spine upright and
   suspend the *Baihui* Point.

   Pull in the chin, shut the lips and
   touch the tongue tip to the teeth ridge.

   Drop the upper eyelids,
   permitting the eye to look forward.

   Tuck in the chest and relax the waist
   as well as the hips.

   Keep both of the elbows outward
   to form hollowed armpits.

   Pull in the stomach and lift the anus
   without any strain.

   Bend the knees, turn them outward
   and then inward for a round crotch.

   Stand firm with feet flat
   and weight evenly distributed.

   For the posture, attention is paid to

softness, roundness and farness.

Explanation

The essentials of the body position of this pattern fall on "roundness and softness". Roundness brings about the free flowing of vital energy and softness can prevent stiffness. The specific method is as follows: Stand firmly with feet flat. Bend the knees slightly. Turn the knees first outward and then inward. Return to the original position, thus bringing about a round crotch. Sink the vital energy and drop the seat slightly to make the hips relaxed. Avoid using effort when pulling in the stomach and lifting the anus. Once the thought reaches these points, the result will be fine. To tuck in the chest refers to pulling in slightly that part of the chest above the pit of the stomach, avoiding any forward thrust of the chest. The back of the body will be lifted when the spine stands erect. It is somewhat contradictory to drop the shoulders and hollow the armpits at the same time, but so long as your attention is paid to the slight out-turning of the elbows, you will get hollow armpits and dropped shoulders. To get the head suspended, you should avoid lifting the head with a stiff neck. When the chin is slightly tucked in, the Point of *Baihui* will face the sky, so the breath can flow freely. Closed eyes help prevent the leakage of vital energy and shuteyes help prevent the dispersing of vital energy. To make the tongue touch the upper palate means to let the tip of the tongue touch the upper teeth ridge. Do not use effort, otherwise, the tongue will get stiff and sore. Swallow the saliva, if there is any, slowly and gradually as if it were sinking into *Dantian*—the Point of *Qihai* (located at about 1.5 *cun* below the navel). For this posture, see figure 21.

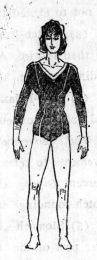

Figure 21

Note: The Pithy Formula starts from the top and goes downward while the Explanation starts from bottom and goes up. To perform it, you should start from bottom to the top and check it up by mental activities from the top to the bottom. By doing this, it helps get quiescence and the vital energy can go down after going up.

Detailed Movements

The Relaxed and Quiescent Form in Standing Position can also be called the Standing *Qigong* Technique. This form of *Qigong* exercise requires a quiescent head, so it's best for you to think of nothing when performing it. If you fail to do so, you can think of the detailed movements of this *Qigong* exercise. The general key point of this exercise is that the whole body is relaxed and free from stiffness. This form of *Qigong* exercise can be divided into 18 detailed steps:

(1) Stand with feet flat and spaced as wide as shoulder width. Keep the feet parallel. Bear the body weight on the point where the feet are perpendicular to the tibae, a point about 2 *cun* inward from the heels.

(2) Knee-Bending: Bend the knees slightly. Your knees

are not to exceed the toe tips.

(3) Crotch-Rounding: Turn both knees first outward and then inward. After that, return to the preceding knee-bending position. This is called "crotch-rounding".

(4) Hip-Relaxing: Drop the seat slightly with the vital energy sunken and the hips will be relaxed.

The above-mentioned four items are the detailed movements to relax the lower limbs in the relaxed and quiescent Qigong exercise in standing position, of which "crotch-rounding" is the key point.

(5) Stomach-Contracting: "Stomach" here refers to the lower part of the abdomen above the pubic bone. When pulling in the stomach, just pull inward the lower part of the abdomen. Do not contract it with force.

(6) Anus-Lifing: Draw in the anus and lift it gently only by mental intention. Do not raise it with effort.

(7) Waist-Relaxing: The relaxing of the waist is very important. It must be performed on the basis of the relaxing of the hips. First stretch the back and then breathe out. And now you will feel the waist relaxed. There are quite a number of ways to relax the waist (head-suspending and chin-tucking-in can also help the waist relax), but it takes a long time for you to make the sacral bone loose.

(8) Chest-Tucking-in: Make the stomach pit cave in. Turn both elbows outward.

(9) Back-Stretching: Straighten up the spine and you will have a sense, in a way, of the opening of the scapula.

These five items mentioned above are the requirements

for the relaxation of the body trunk, of which the relaxation of the waist is the key point.

(10) Shoulder-Drooping: Relax the shoulders and there will be a sensation of the drooping of the upper arms.

(11) Elbow-Dropping: There seems to be something hanging from the elbows.

(12) Wrist-Relaxing: With the fingers down, the wrists will be free and loose.

(13) Armpit-Hollowing: Turn the tips of the elbows outward with the backs of the hands forward, palms slantly toward the trunk. Though the shoulders are drooped, the armpits are hollowed as if they can hold an egg each.

The above-mentioned four items are the essentials of the upper limbs in the quiescent and relaxed standing position, of which "hollow-armpits" is the key point.

(14) Head-Suspending: The *Baihui* Point on the top of the head is perpendicular to the sky (*Baihui* is located in the middle of the line joining the two tips of the ears). When the head is suspended, the head seems to be hanging on a thread.

(15) Cheek-Hooking: In fact this is a necessary step to suspend the head. The head can never get suspended if the chin is not tucked in. When the chin is pulled in, nasal breathing will be free.

(16) Eye-Shutting: Drop the upper eyelids, permitting a thin beam of light (In terms of *Qigong* it is called "to draw the curtains"). This will help the eyes relax. A complete shutting of the eyes will cause tension in the

eyes.

(17) Lip-Closing: Close the lips slightly.

(18) The Tongue Touching the Upper Palate: The tongue touches the upper teeth ridge gently. Do not use force. Only touch the tongue to the teeth ridge.

These five items are the requirements of the head in the relaxed and quiescent standing of *Qigong* exercise, of which head-suspending is the key point.

Of the 18 principles for the relaxed and quiescent *Qigong* exercise in standing position, head-supending, armpit-hollowing, waist-relaxing, and crotch-rounding are the four key points. Among them the relaxation of the waist is the leading factor. So in this exercise, emphasis is on the relaxation of the waist. Without the relaxation of the waist, vital energy can not sink into *Dantian*.

The length of time for relaxed and quiescent *Qigong* exercise in standing position is flexible. If you can reach the stage of relaxation and quiescence in three or five minutes, you are ready for the next form of *Qigong* exercise. The exercise can also last for 20-30 minutes.

2. The Three Deep Exhaling and Inhaling Form

Pithy Formula

With one hand on top of the other at *Dantian*,
    breathe out and in evenly and slowly.
Crouch slightly while breathing out;
    remain crouched when breathing in.
Stand up only after slowly breathing in,
    when the air can flow freely.

Explanation

Make the *Laogong* Point (P. 8) in the inner part of the left hand face *Qihai* (i. e., *Dantian*). Put the right hand on top of the left hand (for females, the right hand under the left hand) (see Figure 22). Breathe out slowly, i. e., to breathe deeply. The breath must be gentle, thin, even and long. In ancient times, the method was called "Slow and Deep Exhaling". Crouch when breathing out through the mouth. Move the tongue from the upper teeth ridge to the lower teeth ridge while crouching. After a short pause, the tongue returns to the upper teeth ridge, and breathe in through the nose. Do not stand up until you stop breathing in (see Figure 23). Regulate breath freely when standing up. Start for a second round when you resume normal breathing. Do three rounds altogether.

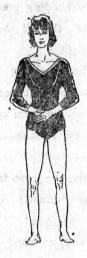

Figure 22

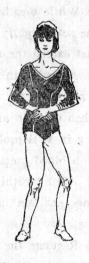

Figure 23

111

Detailed Movements

(1) Start the Three Deep Exhaling and Inhaling Form when the Relaxed and Quiescent Form in Standing Position is over. Before breathing out slowly, put the hands one on top of the other (the right hand on top of the left hand for males, while for females, the left hand on top of the right hand) at *Dantian* below the navel (1.5 *cun* below the navel) with *Yuji* of the thumb placed on the navel and *Laogong* facing *Qihai*.

(2) When breathing out slowly, move the tongue from the upper teeth ridge to the lower teeth ridge. Send out air very slowly and retain a certain leeway. For mental activities, think of letting out completely the turbid substance, or think of the requirements for the softness, thinness, evenness and length, or think of nothing at all.

(3) While breathing out, crouch by bending your knees with the seat slightly lowered until the tips of the knees somewhat exceed the toetips.

(4) After breathing out, stay in the crouching positon and do not stand up. Move your tongue to the upper teeth ridge, then draw in air through the nose. To stand up while breathing in will probably cause tightness in the chest or even high blood pressure.

(5) After breathing in, start to raise the torso from the crouching position and then breathe normally (natural breathing).

(6) Regulate the breath and then start a second round.

(7) Do the third round. When the torso is raised, start

the next pattern of *Qigong* exercise.

3. The Three Open-and-Close Form

Pithy Formula

Start with hands one upon the other over *Dantian*,

and move the hands sidewise, back to back,

till they are half *chi* away from the hips.

Palm facing palm, return them to where they were, and

something is gained from both "open" and "close".

With pathogenic evils out and vital energy in,

you'd better keep *Dantian* closed.

Explanation

When performing the "open-and-close" exercise, carelessness must be avoided. Move the hands inward gently and slowly from off the hips in the figure of arc. For beginners breathing may not be involved. When you have grasped the basic skill, breathe out when "opening" and breathe in when "closing". For mental acitivities, think of the vast plain when you "open" and think of the vital energy's returning to *Dantian* when you "close".

Detailed Movements

(1) Start from the preceding position. Turn the hands back to back at *Dantian*. Move the hands sidewise toward the side of the hips with palms facing outward. This is called the "open form" (See Figure 24).

(2) When performing this starting form, point the fingers to the front (the small finger across the thumb). Move the palms along a horizontal line at the level of *Dantian* until they are about half a *chi* away from the hips.

(3) Turn the palms in an arc to face inward (i. e., facing the centre of the body). With thumbs up and small fingers down, move the hands inward to the central line of the body (see Figure 25) until the fingers of both hands meet. This is called the "close form". Repeat three times.

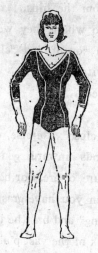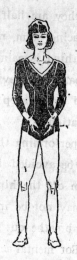

Figure 24   Figure 25

(4) To do this "open" and "close" form, beginners may not involve breathing. When you have practised for some time, you may consider breathing. Breathe out when "opening" and breathe in when "closing". Exhale through the mouth when "opening" and inhale through the nose when "closing".

(5) When doing this form of exercise, you can think either of the actions or of nothing at all. When you are skilled, you can imagine: When opening, it is spacious so that the exogenous pathogenic factors can be expelled, and when closing it is sealed so that the exogenous pathogenic factors

can not get in.

II. Closing Form

You must do the closing form when you are through with a form of *Qigong* exercise. To do the closing form is just like to do the starting form, only in a reverse sequence. That is, to do the Three Open-and-Close Form first, then the Three Deep Exhaling and Inhaling, and finally do the Relaxed and Quiescent Form in Standing Position. The purpose of doing the closing form is to bring the internal energy released through *Qigong* exercise back into *Dantian*. As the saying goes: "Doing *Qigong* exercise without a closing form means to have thrown away what you have gained."

In ancient China, saliva was called "gold fluid" or "jade fluid" and was always considered as treasure, so swallow the saliva down slowly whenever there is any.

Chapter 2
Basic Patterns of *Qigong* Exercise

I. The Breath-Regulating and *Qi*-Reenforcing Pattern

1. The Rudimentary Method to Strengthen Health

Pithy Formula

This method to strengthen health is a rudimentary exercise;

step forward with the heels gently touching the

ground.

Relax your head and waist when waving your arms, looking to the left and right as if in flowering shrubs.

In flowering shrubs, you walk leisurely, with a smile on your face and light at heart.

If you ask: "How do I breathe?"

breathe through the nasal cavity like blowing wind.

Explanation

The Health-strengthening Method is an exercise of free style. You will gain your goal so long as you keep walking with the heels touching the ground, keep to the requirements of the Relaxed and Quiescent Form in Standing Position: press your tongue against the upper teeth ridge with a smile on your face; turn your head and the waist, with the arms swinging gently. When skilled in walking, start blowing in and out slowly through the nasal cavity.

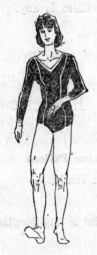

Detailed Movements

(1) Start from the Relaxed and Quiescent Form in Standing Position. Step forward, with the right foot first and then with the left foot, the heel touching the ground. When walking, keep the feet at shoulder width, as in standing position(see Figure 26).

(2) When stepping forward, just walk as you usually do. Don't

Figure 26

oversway your arms. Try to be natural.

(3) The arms swing with the turning of the waist.

(4) The turning of the waist is guided by the turning of the head.

(5) Breathe in and out through the nasal cavity.

(6) You should be self-possessed, light-hearted, happy and relaxed. Imagine you have walked into some flowering shrubs, looking to the right and to the left, and there are so many beautiful things that you can hardly take them all in. Therefore, there should be a smile on your face, or at least a touch of smile. To smile is also a sort of *Qigong* technique.

2. The Fixed-Step Blowing Method

Pithy Formula

The Fixed-Step Blowing Method has nine steps for
each leg;
keep the key points in mind and relax the waist.
To step out with the right foot first to reenforce vital
energy;
the toe tip touches the ground and the foot falls flat.
Keep the heel firm whem the toetip is raised, and
move the hands up and down obviously.
The head guides the waist to rotate, covering three
directions;
inhale and exhale gently and evenly through the nose.
Weight shifts to the right when the turning is to the left;
hold the right foot firm and flat when the left heel is
lifted.

With the neck relaxed, the spine will straighten up;

and with the waist turning, the lumbar vertebra will be loosened.

Swing from the left to the right;

the key points are the same as when performed in reverse.

Explanation

The Fixed-Step Blowing Method is the preparatory step of the Breath-Regulating and Qi-Reenforcing Pattern. Step out with the right foot, toetip touching the ground, and then place it flat on the ground; raise the toetip with the heel remaining on the ground. With the hands slightly lifted, and palms facing each other, the left arm swings leftward, which is followed by the right arm. At the same time, the neck guides the waist to turn from the right to the left. The neck leads the waist in turning and the waist leads the arms in swinging. Inhale twice through the nose while the right foot is being placed flat, and exhale once while the left foot is being lifted. To inhale and exhale through the nose is called the Blowing Method. Shift the body weight onto the right foot after blowing. When the whole body is relaxed, put down the left foot and distribute the weight evenly on both feet, with arms swinging naturally. Now the first round of the Fixed-Step Blowing Method is ended. Do this nine times altogether with the right foot in the front. Then move the left foot forward and return to the relaxed and quiescent standing position and do the open-and-close exercise three times. Now, step out with the left foot and begin the

118

left-side Fixed-Step Blowing Method. The direction is changed but the principles are the same. Do this nine times as well.

Detailed Movements

(1) Start the Fixed-Step Blowing Method, hands at your sides. Step out with the right foot, and place it flat immediately after the tip touches the ground, then lift the tip up (see Figure 27).

(2) Turn the torso to the left naturally with the weight on the left foot.

(3) Drop the seat slightly and lower the waist, with the back leg bent and the front leg relaxed, turn the waist to the right. Swing both arms to the right until the left hand reaches the midline and the right hand reaches the right side of the hip; turn the head to the right, eyes looking to the right (see Figure 28).

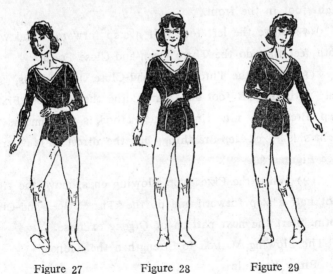

Figure 27   Figure 28   Figure 29

(4) Turn the waist to the left, and shift the weight from the left to the right. Swing both hands from the right to the left until the left hand reaches the left hip, and the right hand reaches the midline; turn the head from the right to the front, and then to the left, eyes looking in the same directions (see Figure 29).

(5) Shift the weight from the left to the right heel, inhale twice (through the nose), place the right foot flat and lift the left heel; bend the front leg and relax the back leg(now the right hand reaches the midline). Inhale once through the nose.

(6) Swing both hands naturally toward the right, shift the weight to the right, and raise the right tiptoe again. This is the end of the first round of the Fixed -Step Blowing Method. Do nine times altogether with the right foot in the front.

(7) Move the left foot half a step forward; stand with both feet flat; do the Three Open-and-Close Form.

(8) When the Three Open-and-Close Form ends, step out with the left foot and start doing the left-side Fixed-step Breathing nine times. The method is the same as the right-side Fixed-step Breathing, but the direction is reversed (See Figures 30—32).

(9) When the Fixed-step Blowing ends, move the right foot half a step forward and do the Three Open-and-Close Form. Start the next pattern of Qigong exercise.

3. The Blowing Method to Strengthen the Kidney

Pithy Formula

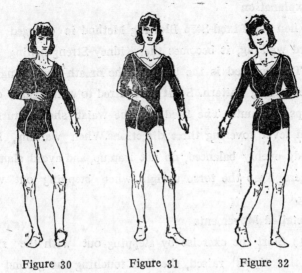

Figure 30   Figure 31   Figure 32

Kidney strengthening is a basic pattern that
    reenforces the primordial *Qi* and the essence of life.
Concentrate the thought on the tiptoe with the toe raised,
    and when the thought reaches the gate of life,
        there's a sense of lightness in the lower limbs.
Inhale twice for one step and exhale once for another
    step, and draw in and send out air like the wind
    blowing.
The head leads the waist in turning,
    and the arms move with the waist.
The backbone is relaxed when the head is suspended, and
    the kidney-energy rises with the turning of the waist.
The mind and the vital energy are in harmony, and
    the blood and *Qi* flow freely along the channels and
    collaterals.

Explanation

When the Fixed-Step Blowing Method is changed into forward walking, it becomes the Kidney-Strengthening Method. This method is the basis of the Breath-Regulating and Qi-Reenforcing Pattern. So it is required to walk faster, over 60 steps a minute. The head and the waist should turn at a fixed level covering three directions.When walking, keep the body evenly balanced, do not leap up, and avoid slanting shoulders. Keep the torso upright when stepping out with the leg.

Detailed Movements

(1) Start the exercise by stepping out with the right foot, the tiptoe raised, the heel touching the ground (see Figure 33).

(2) When stepping out with the left foot, also raise the tiptoe and touch the ground with the heel (see Figure 34).

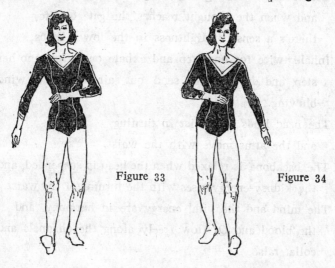

Figure 33   Figure 34

(3) Turn the head from the right, to the front, and then back to the right, covering three directions in a fan shape.

(4) Do the exercise with eyes open. (A beam of light is permitted when the upper eyelids drop.)

(5) The waist turns with the head. The hips do not turn.

(6) The turning of the waist brings the arms into action. When stepping out with the right foot, the left arm moves down to Dantian from the heart pit, and then goes toward the direction of the left hip. The right hand moves from the right towards the midline of the torso as well as the heart pit with palms tilted toward the body; shift the body weight from the left to the right.

(7) While stepping out with the left foot, move the right hand from the heart pit towards Dantian and then in the direction of the right hip. Move the left hand from the left towards the heart pit at the midline of the torso. Shift the weight from the right to the left.

(8) When swinging the arms, the maximum angle between each arm and the torso should not exceed 60 degrees.

(9) When stepping out with the right foot, inhale twice through the nose; exhale once through the nose when stepping out with the left foot.

(10) While doing this exercise, concentrate the thoughts on the toe tips so that the heel can touch the ground gently and smoothly, which helps prevent pain. Thoughts concen-

trated on the heel can cause pain in the heel.

(11) When you are skilled in walking, if you can not calm yourself down when doing the exercise, use the Breath-Listening Method. That is, listen to the sounds of inhaling and exhaling through the nose, so as to get rid of distracting thoughts.

(12) Another way leading to quiescence: When looking in the three directions, look in such a way that everything seems indistinct, as if there were nothing around you and you could see nothing though you are looking.

(13) When walking, keep the feet at shoulder width, as in standing position, and move forward along an S-shape line (but the feet are kept parallel). Walk 60—70 steps a minute.

4. The Blowing Method to Strengthen the Lung, the Spleen and the Kidney

Pithy Formula

Foot-touching and finger-twisting transmitted to three channels,
    walk forward with toetip touching the ground once every step.
Twist the *Shaoshang* Point with the forefingers,
    sending a message to the Lung Channel of Hand *Taiyin*.
Touch the ground with the tip of the big toe,
    to arouse the Liver and Spleen Channels of Foot-*yin*.
Toe-touching and hand-twisting take place simultaneously,

accompanied in harmony by nasal breathing.

Inhale twice through the nose when stepping out,

the left foot and the right foot alternate off and on.

Explanation

The Method to Strengthen the Lung, the Spleen and the Kidney was originally divided into three methods, but they were similar in the foot's touching the ground. Besides, the foot-touching is accompanied by finger-twisting, so the repeated actions are very hard to distinguish. The combination of the three makes the performance easier and brings about no harm. When stepping out with the right foot, inhale twice through the nose with the hands swinging from the right to the left. When they reach the side of the right shoulder, hold the left foot straight up with toes down to touch the ground. Meanwhile, rub the *Shaoshang* Point on the thumbs with the forefingers and exhale through the nose. The three movements are performed harmoniously. After the left foot touches the ground, step out with it. Then touch the ground with the right tiptoe similarly, but the direction is the opposite (Note: Do not rotate the heel when the tiptoe touches the ground).

Detailed Movements

The basic technique of this method is the same as that of the Method to Strengthen the Kidney. Its differences are as follows:

(1) Step out with the right foot, both hands moving in the same pose. After inhaling twice through the nose, step out with the left foot. When stepping out with the left

foot, give the ground a touch with the tiptoe instead of touching the ground with the heel(see Figure 35).

(2) When the tiptoe touches the ground, both hands are on the left side of the body with fingers bent as if to grasp. The thumbs and the forefingers rub each other at the *Shaoshang* Point(at the root of the nail on the inner part of the thumb) and the *Shaoyang* Point (at the root of the nail on the inner part of the forefinger). (see Figure 36)

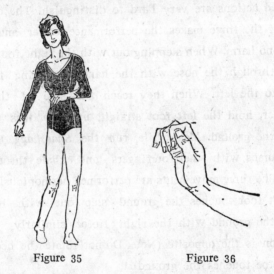

Figure 35   Figure 36

(3) Exhale through the nose when the tiptoe touches the ground and the fingers rub each other.

(4) Step out with the left foot immediately after its tip touches the ground. Then the heel of the left foot falls onto the ground and inhale twice through the nose.

(5) The right tiptoe touches the ground with the two hands on the right side of the body rubbing the *Shaoshang*

and *Shaoyang* points. Meanwhile exhale twice throuth the nose.

(6) Step out with the right foot, the heel touching the ground. Inhale twice through the nose....Go on repeating this. An appropriate pace is 50—60 steps a minute.

5. The Blowing Method to Strengthen the Heart

Pithy Formula (1)

The Blowing Method to Strengthen the Heart is a four-step exercise.

The first three steps are accompanied with breathing but the fourth step is not.

Inhale on the right step and on the left step as well, and

exhale like wind blowing when moving the right foot forward again.

Both middle fingers touch the *Laogong* on the fourth step,

and there seems to be a sound though no breathing.

The rubbing of the forefingers takes place only on the left steps, and

the two feet move onward without stopping.

Swing the arms gently during the performance,

with a light heart and a quiescent, empty head.

Pithy Formula (2)

The heart-strengthening method has 4 inhalations and 3 exhalations,

the key-point of the exercise is the rubbing of *Zhongchong.*

Inhale 4 times in succession on both the right step and
the left step;

inhale twice on the right step and hold the breath on
the left step.

Both arms swing gently from the left to the
right;

the empty and quiescent head thinks of nothing.

Walk and perform gently and slowly;

don't forget to accompany the performance with
breathing.

Explanation

Two methods of heart-strengthening are introduced
here. The former is easy to perform and the latter
is benefitial to the circulation of vital energy along the *Ren*
Channel and the *Du* Channel. Each method has its own
characteristics and both have remarkable effects. The key
points of the Blowing Method to Strengthen the Heart are
to obtain quiescence of the mind and smooth flow of the
Qi. Both methods have four continuous steps. Rub the
Zhongchong Point against the *Laogong* Point on the palm.

Detailed Movements (for Pithy Formula 1)

(1) This method is based on the Method to Strengthen
the Kidney. Four steps make a unit. Inhale on the first
step; inhale again on the second step; exhale on the third
step; (all through the nose); hold the breath on the fourth
step. (See Figure 37)

(2) For the first step, move the right foot out and
inhale when the heel touches the ground; start the second

128

step by moving the left foot out and inhale when its heel touches the ground; for the third step, step out with the right foot and exhale when the heel touches the ground; hold the breath on the fourth step. This is repeated again and again.

(3) When holding the breath on the fourth step, both hands are on the left side of the body, the *Zhongchong* Point of the middle finger touching the *Laogong* Point of the palm. (If you fail to touch the *Laogong* Point, you can touch any point on the palm.) (see Figure 38)

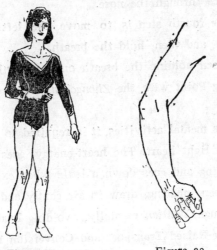

Figure 37   Figure 38

(4) Except for the touching of the *Zhongchong* Point on the fourth step, the swinging of the hands is the same as that of the Method to Strengthen the Kidney, but the span of movement is smaller with an angle between the arms and the torso limited to about 30 degrees. The pace of walking

is limited to appropriately 45 steps per minute.

(5) The heart should be calm and the mind quiescent.
Detailed Movements (for Pithy Formula 2)

(1) This method, based on the Method to Strengthen the Kidney, also has four steps as a unit.

(2) Inhale twice in succession through the nose when stepping out with the right foot.

(3) Inhale twice through the nose when stepping out with the left foot.

(4) For the third step, move the right foot out and exhale twice through the nose.

(5) The fourth step is to move the left foot out and exhale once, and then, hold the breath.

(6) When holding the breath on the fourth step, touch the *Laogong* Point with the *Zhongchong* Point of the middle finger.

(7) For mental activities, it is required to have a happy mind and a light heart. The heart-energy goes up slightly when inhaling and goes down a little when exhaling.

(8) When inhaling, draw in air gently and bit by bit. Inhale through *Dantian* mentally, avoiding loud noise.

Ⅱ. The Toe-Raised Transport and Conversion Pattern

This essential *Qigong* pattern joins the left with the right and communicates the upper to the lower. It regulates the heart, the breath and the physical body, through which run the key elements of *Qigong*. Attention should be paid to both motion and quiescence; any partiality should be avoided. All the three *Dantians* are considered but the turbidity and the clarity should be distinguished. The vital energy circulates automatically in the body, and *daoyin* and *anqiao* are involved in walking.

1. The Open-and-Close Method at the Three *Dantians*

   Pithy Formula

   The Open-and-Close Method at the Three *Dantians*
   has a most stable curative effect.
   Step out half a step with the right foot,
   and bring the hands to *Dantian*.
   Raise them up to *Yingtang*, and
   join the palms with fingers pointing to the sky.
   Bend the fingers a little when closing,
   and turn the palms out when opening.
   Set the hands apart, wider than shoulder width,
   and pay attention to the roundness of the elbows.
   Have the palms facing each other when closing,
   and move the hands slowly toward the upper *Dantian*.
   Bend the palms slightly when lowering the hands,
   and at *Dantian* the fingertips touch each other.
   When the hands reach the middle *Dantian*,
   do "open-and-close" once more.
   The trunk is bent and drawn back now and then,
   with the weight shifting from the back to the front.
   When the third open-and-close starts,
   the exhalation takes place at the lower *Dantian*.
   Lower the back leg when crouching,
   and keep the waist upright.
   Crouch like a landing goose,

and stand up carefree and leisurely.

Open and close at the three *Dantians*,

   each time with a horizontal movement.

Shift the body weight to the key-points;

   raise and drop the hands at the *Shanzhong* Point.

Perform once, facing each of the four directions,

   altogether 8 times clockwise and counter-clockwise.

Breathe naturally from beginning to end;

   the steady flow of *Qi* brings about a clear mind.

Exhale when opening and inhale when closing, and

   the *Qi* will be even and smooth.

Explanation

   The Open-and-Close Method at the Three *Dantians* means to do the open-and-close exercise once at each of the following three points horizontally: *Yintang*—the Upper *Dantian*, *Qihai*—the Middle *Dantian*, and *Huiyin*—the Lower *Dantian*. The specific method is as follows: Step out half a step with the right foot, arms hanging down and fingertips slightly bent. Move the hands up from the abdomen, just alongside the *Ren* Channel, keeping the hands half a *chi* away from the abdomen and the chest (see Figure 39—40). Turn the fingertips up when they reach *Yingtang*, keeping the *Laogong* Point and the brows at the same level. At the same time, shift the weight onto the right foot so that the left foot becomes weightless. At *Yingtang* make the hands hollow and move them inward (see Figure 41). Then turn the palms out, back to back, and do the "open" movement (see Figure 42), avoiding the posture of "surrender" and

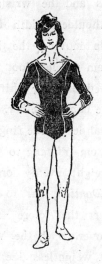

Figure 39

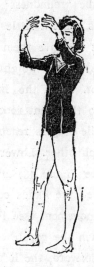

Figure 40

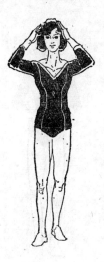

Figure 41

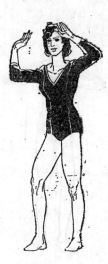

Figure 42

keeping the "roundness" of the elbows and the wrists. Set the hands apart a little wider than shoulder width before you start to move them inward. While moving the hands inward, shift the weight gradually from the left foot to the right foot. When the hands are moved inward, shift the weight to the right foot and bring the hands together. When the middle fingers reach the horizontal level, the fingertips touch each other. Lower the hands from *Yintang* to *Shanzhong* (see Figure 43) and keep the weight evenly on both feet. When the hands come down to *Dantian*, start to do the "open" movement (see Figure 44). Start the "close" movement when the "open" movement is over. With the weight shifted forward, the left foot becomes weightless (see Figure 45—46). After the "close" movement, raise both hands in an arc to *Shanzhong*. Lower the hands and crouch to a

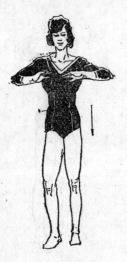

Figure 43

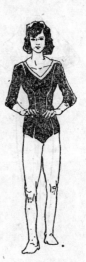

Figure 44

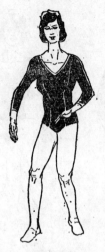
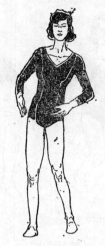

Figure 45   Figure 46

position where the thigh of the front leg becomes flat. (Those
who have leg trouble, crouch slightly and have the hands
performing in concert with *Huiyin*.) Do the open-and-close
in front of the horizontal leg at the level of *Huiyin*.
Distribute the weight on both foot, with the front one
bearing a little more than the back one. Meanwhile, avoid
any bending of the upper body or lowering of the head (see
Figure 47—49). Stand up when the open-and-close at the
Lower *Dantian* is over. When standing up, rise slowly with
hands hanging down naturally just like the morning sun
gradually coming out of the waters. After standing up, raise
the hands to *Shanzhong* with weight distributed on both
feet. Drop the hands down to *Dantian* in a manner slightly
open (see Figure 50). Then the left foot turns 90 degrees
(see Figure 51) and the torso turns with it. Hold the right

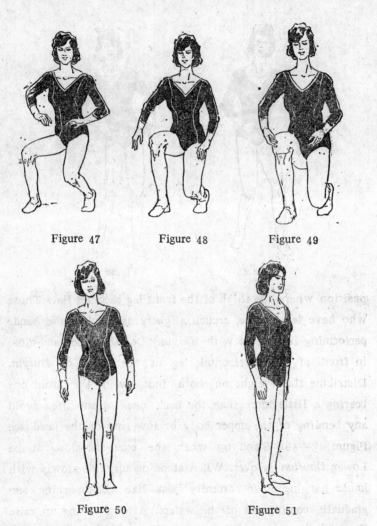

Figure 47   Figure 48   Figure 49

Figure 50   Figure 51

heel weightless and move a step forward with the right foot
still in the front(see Figure 52—53). Do this four times,
turning in the opposite direction of the path of the sun.
When you have finished doing it in the fourth direction,

136

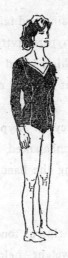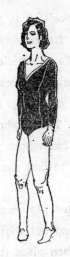

Figure 52   Figure 53

step out with the left foot, remain at the original place, and do the open-and-close at the three *Dantians* four times in the same direction as the sun's path. The specific methods are the same as mentioned above, except that the left foot is in the front. When the fifth open-and-close at the three *Dantians* is finished, turn 90 degrees with the tiptoe as the axis and the body turns with it. Go on performing in this direction until the second four rounds of open-and-close at the three *Dantians* are over.

Now the Open-and-Close Method at the Three *Dantians* —a preparation form of the Toe-Raised Transport and Conversion Pattern, is over. By now the left foot is in front of the right, which suits the beginning of the next pattern of *Qigong* exercise.

In the Open-and-Close Method at the Three *Dantians*,

the hand position is very important. Rising and falling with palms and fingers downwards can treat hyperactivity of *yang* which leads to deficiency of *yin*, e. g. high blood pressure, while with the palms upwards, can treat diseases due to the deficiency of *yang*, e. g. low blood pressure and low hemogram. Those who have no deficiency or hyperactivity problems, but whose *yin* and *yang* are unbalanced, can keep the palms toward the body when moving the hands up and down.

Detailed Movements

(1) Step out with the right foot, tiptoe touching the ground. Then place it flat with the weight held in the middle of the two legs.

(2) Bring the hands together in front of the Middle *Dantian*.

(3) Move both hands upward alongside the Midline of the abdomen. Those who have the problem of hyperactivity of *yang* which leads to the deficiency of *yin*, can raise the hands a little bit faster with fingers pointing downward (see Figure 54).

For those who are weak and easy to get tired due to deficiency of *yang*, move the hands slowly upwards with the palms facing up (see Figure 55).

Those who have no deficiency or hyperactivity problems, but whose *yin* and *yang* are unbalanced, raise the hands at the normal pace with fingers pointing to each other (see Figure 56).

(4) After the hands reach the level of *Shanzhong*, the

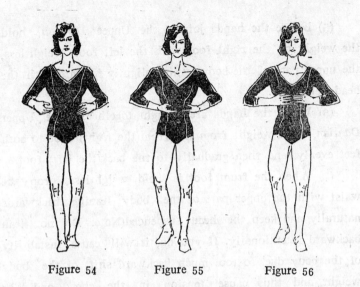

| Figure 54 | Figure 55 | Figure 56 |

hand position changes with the changing of the body position. For example, with the moving up of the hands, you first turn the fingers originally pointing downwards to point at each other, and gradually you turn them to point upwards, and then, you join the palms at the Upper *Dantian* (*Yintang*, a point between the brows). So, for fingers originally pointing to each other, turn them upward and bring them together, palm to palm, at the Upper *Dantian*; and for palms facing upwards originally, turn the fingers gradually to point at each other when they have reached the level of *Shanzhong*, and then, with the fingers pointing upwards, join the palms at the Upper *Dantian*. When moving up the hands, avoid square shoulders or bent fingers pointing at the chest or the neck. Otherwise it would cause tightness in the chest, nausea and dizziness.

(5) Before the hands join at the Upper *Dantian*, hold the weight on the right foot with the left foot weightless, the upper part of the body leaning slightly forward with the head held erect.

(6) When the hands are brought together at the Upper *Dantian*, shift weight from the front(the right) foot to both feet evenly, and then gradually to the back(the left) foot.

(7) When the front foot is held weightless, drop the waist with the upper part of the body leaning backwards naturally and keep the head suspended(Note: Do not lean backward intentionally. If you do, it will cause instability of the body due to too much backward shift of the body weight, and thus cause tension in the chest and the heart.)

(8) When doing the "open" movement, change the hands from palm to palm to back to back. With the weight shifted backward, move both hands outwards in an arc alongside the horizontal level of *Yintang*. Part them a little wider than shoulder width. Keep the fingers of both hands, the palms, and the arms in a round arc in line with the upper part of the chest. Keep the shoulders and elbows dropped, too. If you have difficulty in doing so, you should do it mentally.

(9) Keep the *Laogong* Point in line with the *Yintang* Point at the horizontal level when doing the "open" movement.

(10) When you change the opening motion into the closing motion, bring the hands together at *Yintang*, palm

to palm. In the course of closing, shift the body weight from the back foot to the front foot, thus, the upper part of the body leaning naturally forward.

(11) When the closing movement is over and the hands have dropped to the Point of *Shanzhong*, distribute the weight evenly on both feet. There are three forms of hand-dropping:

① For those who have the problem of hyperactivity of *yang*, point the fingertips toward each other and move the hands down slowly. The speed of hand-dropping is slower than that of hand-rising.

② For those who are weak and easily get tired due to the deficiency of *yang*, connect the fingertips and move the hands down, palm to palm, comparatively faster alongside the chest.

③ For those whose even balance between *yin* and *yang* has broken down, turn the palms inward (toward the body) when the fingertips are touching each other. The speed of hand-dropping is the same as that of hand-rising.

(12) Do the open-and-close form when the hands reach the Middle *Dantian*. The weight is held on the back foot when opening, while closing, the weight is held on the front foot. The rest of the movements are the same as those of the open-and-close exercise at the Upper *Dantian*.

(13) When you are through with the open-and-close movements, raise the hands to *Shanzhong*. Place the feet flat and hold the weight on both feet before you go on to move the hands downward. (There are also three forms of

hand-dropping and hand-rising.)

(14) When the hands move downward after surpassing
Dantian, crouch simultaneously. Have the heels raised
naturally and the weight distributed on both feet with the
front foot bearing a little more. The purpose of squatting
down is to let the hands do open-and-close in front of
the knees at the Lower *Dantian* (*Huiyin*).

(15) Stand up when the open-and-close at the Lower
Dantian is over. With the rising of the body the hands rise
naturally. Do not purposely raise them. After standing up,
raise the hands to the level of *Shanzhong*. Then move the
hands downward smoothly, set them slightly apart at the
Middle *Dantian*. Turn the body.

(16) The method of body turning is: turn the back foot
90 degrees and let the body turn with it. The front foot
becomes the back foot. If you were facing the east, now you
are facing the north after the turn.

(17) Step out with the back foot to change it into the
front foot. The right foot is still in the front. Now start a
second round of open-and-close at the three *Dantians*.

(18) Do the Open-and-Close at the Three *Dantians* once
at each of the four directions: the east, the north, the west
and the south; four rounds altogether.

(19) When you are through with the four rounds of
Open-and-Close at the Three *Dantians*, start another four
rounds in the opposite direction, i. e., the south, the west,
the north and the east. Perform it with the left foot in the
front. The rest movements are the same as when performing

with the right foot in the front.

(20) When the reverse four rounds of Open-and-Close at the Three *Dantians* are over, you will find yourself facing the same direction in which you started. So when you choose the direction for the first open-and-close, you should consider a direction suitable for the next pattern of exercise, when all the open-and-close exercises at the three *Dantians* are finished.

(21) When performing the open-and-close exercise, you may not do the breathing exercise at the same time. You can breathe naturally. When you are skilled, you may exhale slowly when opening and inhale when closing. But you should not do the breathing exercise when you do the open -and-close exercise at the Lower *Dantian*.

(22) For mental activities of the first stage in the open-and-close at the three *Dantians*, concentrate your mind on the movements themselves, but when you are skilled, you'd better think of nothing (with a quiescent mind). If you fail to get a quiescent mind, you may count at heart, e.g. one for "rise", two for "open", three for "close", four for "fall" .... You can make up your own numerals.

2. The Toe-Raised Slow Walking Method
   Pithy Formula
   The previous exercise ends
      with the left foot in the front.
   The head leads the waist in turning
      with the right hand first in motion.

When the left hand reaches *Shangwan*,
    step out with the right foot naturally.
Shift the weight to the left foot,
    and make the right weightless and at ease.
Gently the heel touches the ground,
    which is followed by the external foot edge.
All the five toes press down on the ground,
    the waist is turned leftward.
Raise the right hand to *Shangwan* and
    guide the fingers of the left hand to *Weizhong*.
Waist relaxed, hips dropped and the vital energy
    returned,
    the body weight is still shifted to the right
    side.
Step out with the right foot at the start, and
    the key points are the same as those of the previous
    exercise.
Walk slowly like floating clouds,
    like water flowing in a stream.
This exercise is mental, and
    relaxation and concentration are essential.
Silent counting replaces all thoughts, and
    there is no thinking—nothing at all.
Keep the nine-step *daoyin* in mind and
    relax, but do not slack, and the channels will be
    dredged.
The head leads the waist in turning, while
    the spirit guides the vital energy.

Walk slowly, naturally and comfortably, and
    the transported and converted spleen-energy fills the
    viscera.
A quiescent mind, free from worries,
    brings forth a good circulation of blood and *Qi*.

Explanation

The keypoints of the Toe-Raised Slow Walking Method
are relaxation and quiescence. That is why it is also called
a "Mental Exercise". When performing, it's a good idea
to count some figures silently to yourself, i. e., to count
for nine steps before you do *daoyin* once. The method of
daoyin is that, after nine steps, you adjust the body to the
upright position and let the hands swing with the body. When
the hands are raised to *Shanzhong*, move the hands downward
along the *Ren* Channel to *Dantian*. Then set the hands
apart naturally and take the advantage of this pose to start
the Toe-Raised Slow Walking Method. In the pithy formula,
it says, "The right foot is weightless and at ease." That is
to say "When the weight is on the foot, it is as firm as if
rooted and when it is weightless, it should be as weightless as
weightless could be." If the weight is held on the left foot,
the right foot should be weightless and at ease. But before
stepping out, you should first place it down firmly on the
ground, and then step out with it. While performing this
exercise, those who have asthenia-syndromes such as low
blood pressure and the ptosis of the viscera, should have
their palms slantly upward during the course of walking
forward, and stop swinging the hands when they reach the

Middle *Dantian.* It is not necessary to raise them to the level of *Shangwan.* When performing this exercise, you may do the "nine-step *daoyin*" nine times, and then start doing the open-and-close exercise at the two *Dantians.* Once you have mastered the key points of this method, you will feel comfortable all over after the exercise.

Detailed Movements

(1) Start from the preceding Open-and-Close Method at the Three *Dantians* (with the left foot in the front), (see Figure 57). First turn the body leftward, hold the right heel weightless and step out with the right foot(see Figure 58). Relax the waist simultaneously and shift the weight to the left (see Figure 59). The head turns toward the left, from the right to the front, and then to the left. The waist turns with the head.

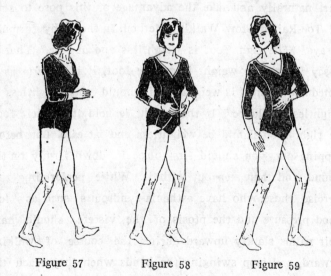

Figure 57   Figure 58   Figure 59

(2) The waist brings the arms into swinging. When the left hand reaches *Shangwan* above the heart pit, the right hand is by the side of the right hip.

(3) To start the walking, step out with the right foot, with the heel touching the ground (see Figure 60)and the tiptoe inwards. Place the whole foot gradually on the ground, first the external edge of the foot, then the small toe, the 4th toe, the 3rd toe, the 2nd toe and the big toe in sequence (see Figure 61). The weight shifts gradually to the right foot and the left foot becomes weightless (see Figure 62).

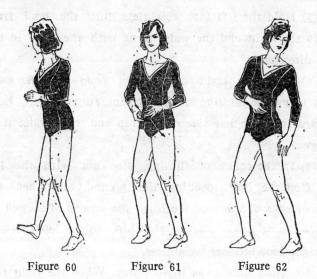

Figure 60　　　　Figure 61　　　　Figure 62

(4) The head turns from the right to the left and simultaneously the waist turns with it.

(5) While the head and the waist are turning leftwards, move the left hand down from *Shangwan* to the side of

the left hip along the Midline and the groin. Move the right hand toward the front from the right side of the hip, and raise it in an arc away from the body until it reaches the *Shangwan* Point. Keep the palms slantly facing the body. For those who suffer from neurasthenia, keep the palms tilted upwards when the hands move up, and keep the palms facing the trunk and *Dantian* when the hands move down. Move the hands like this continuously from the left to right, up and down.

(6) Relax the waist and shift the weight to the right foot.

(7) Hold the left foot weightless, turn the head from left to the right and the waist turns with the head in the same direction.

(8) Move the right hand down from the *Shangwan* Point along the Midline and the groin. Turn the left hand forward from the left side of the hip and then raise it to *Shangwan*.

(9) In the course of turning, step out with the left foot, first the heel touching the ground, and then the external edge of the foot touching the ground, followed by the toes in sequence. The weight shifts to the left foot and the right foot becomes weightless.

(10) Walk nine steps in this way. When the right foot is in front, move the left hand up immediately after it reaches the front of the thigh. And when the right hand reaches the front, do not raise it immediately, let it wait for the left hand and move them up together (see Figure 63). Raise

them to *Shanzhong* and then drop them down to *Dantian*, with palms down, along the Midline of the body (see Figure 64) where they part and move to the left and right hips separately. This movement is called *"daoyin"*. Because there is one *daoyin* in every nine steps, it is also called "nine steps and one *daoyin*".

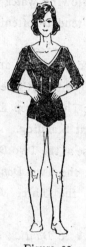

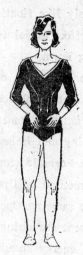

Figure 63   Figure 64

(11) After the *daoyin*, the weight is held on the right foot, the left hand is at the left hip and the right hand is lifted to the *Shangwan* Point .... Start walking again by stepping out with the left foot.

(12) Do one more *daoyin* after nine steps.

(13) This is a mental exercise. While walking, count some figures silently to expel all the distracting thoughts.

(14) The breathing method of Toe-Raised Slow Walking Method is natural breathing.

149

(15) The Toe-Raised Slow Walking Method requires 2-4 steps per minute. For patients of coronary heart diseases and high blood pressure, it is most advisable to walk 2-3 steps per minute, performing 6-9 rounds of "nine steps and one *daoyin*" each time.

(16) This method requires walking slowly and continuously like floating clouds and flowing water so as to gain the effect of joint-loosening, and tendon-softening.

3. Ending Form

The ending form of the Toe-Raised Transport and Conversion Pattern includes four parts: Open-and-Close at the Two *Dantians*, Abdomen-Kneading, the Three Deep Exhaling and Inhaling and Relaxed and Quiescent Standing.

Pithy Formula (for Open-and-Close at the Two *Dantians*)
The method of Open-and-Close at the Two *Dantians* is
   the same as Open-and-Close at the Three *Dantians*
   except crouching.

Vital energy should be guided back to *Dantian* and
   the mind should be free from distracting thoughts.

Pithy Formula (for the Abdomen-Kneading Method)
Place both hands at *Dantian*, one on top of the other, and
   concentrate your mind on *Dantian* soon after you
   calm down.

Knead the abdomen 36 times in a clockwise motion and
   move your hands in small circles which increase to
   large circles.

The lowest point is limited to the pubic symphysis,
   while the highest point may reach the heartpit.

Perform this over the clothes, and

    knead 24 times counter-clockwise frombig circles to

    small circles.

Concentrate all your thoughts on *Dantian*, and

    you will enter a still and quiet world.

Explanation

The starting form of the Self-Controlled *Qigong* Therapy does not require the concentration of thoughts, but requires the regulation of the heart and relaxation. When performing the main part of the exercise, you do not have to concentrate the thoughts on *Dantian*, or on any object in the surroundings, instead, you simply listen to the sound of your own breathing, looking vaguely into the farness and counting some figures silently to yourself, while the Ending Form requires that thoughts should be concentrated on *Dantian*. The abdomen-kneading belongs to the Ending Form, so thoughts should be concentrated on Middle *Dantian*, and silent counting of figures is used for mental activities. When kneading the abdomen, the right hand is placed on top of the left **for** males, while for females, the left hand on top of the right (See Figure 65).

The direction of hand-circling for both males and females, is decided according to the direction of the fingertips of the hand on top. For males, the hands move 36 times clockwise (while for females the hands move counter-clockwise) around *Dantian* from small circles to larger circles limited to *Shanzhong* at the top and the pubis at the bottom. When the 36 circles are over, the hands are just below the *Shanzhong* Point. Change the hands over (for males, put the left hand on top of the right, while for females, the right on top of the left) (see Fingure 66). The

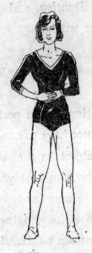
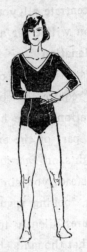

Figure 65   Figure 66

hands move around 24 times in the opposite direction, from larger circles to smaller circles. When you are through with the 24 circles, you'll find your hands at *Dantian* again. Change the hands over and do the Three Deep Exhaling and Inhaling, and the Relaxed and Quiescent Standing as well. Swallow down the saliva (to be swallowed in three portions).

Detailed Movements

(1) Open-and-Close at the Two *Dantian*s is the same as the Openand-Close at the Three *Dantian*s, only it does not require doing the open-and-close at the Lower *Dantian* in squatting position. The mind is concentrated on the gathering of

152

the vital energy toward the Middle *Dantian*. Do this exercise three times. If you fail to concentrate your thoughts on *Dantian*, go on doing this exercise until your thoughts are concentrated on *Dantian*.

(2) The method of Abdomen-Kneading is the same as explained previously.

(3) The Three Deep Exhaling and Inhaling Form is the same as that in the Starting Form.

(4) The Relaxed and Quiescent Standing is the same as that in the Starting Form. Swallow down the saliva in three portions if there is any. When ending the exercise, change both hands into fists, thumbs bent at the inner part of the forefingers, so as to help bring back the vital energy.

(5) When the Relaxed and Quiescent Standing ends, remain standing for 3-5 minutes. Then, open your eyes, withdraw the left foot and walk slowly and leisurely.

(6) The mental activities in the Ending Form begin to change when doing the Open-and-Close at the Two *Dantians*, i. e., the concentration of thoughts on the Middle *Dantian* replaces the silent counting. The mental activities for Abdomen-Kneading are also concentrated on the Middle *Dantian*. After the Ending Form of the Relaxed and Quiescent Standing, stop concentrating thoughts on *Dantian*, and then open your eyes.

III. The Head-Massaging and Mind-Tranquilizing Pattern

1. *Yintang* Point Massage

Pithy Formula

Seat the body firm, and place the legs flat.

The starting Form is necessary for the Sitting Pattern.

Move both hands up to *Yintang*, a point of the Extra Channels.

and the highest point of the three *Dantians*.

With the channels and collaterals uninterrupted,

the mechanism of *Qi* functions well.

Massage can immediately put you in high spirits.

Massage the point leftwards and rightwards with dagger fingers.

For "point respiration" you need calmness.

Explanation

Head-Massage is a combination of the sitting method and the massaging method. Sit on a bench, keeping to the requirements of the Relaxed and Quiescent Standing Form. Choose a bench the hight of which is suitable for you to sit with the legs vertical and the thighs flat. Try to get quiescent after you sit down. When you have calmed down, do the Three Deep Exhaling and Inhaling Form and the Three Open-and-Close Form. Then relax the wrists and move both hands to *Yintang*. Bend the ring finger and small finger with the thumb pressed on top of the ring finger, and put the forefinger across the middle finger—this is called "dagger finger". When both hands have formed dagger fingers, put the tip of the middle finger of the left at the *Yintang* Point, and then place the tip of the middle finger of the right hand at the root of the nail of the left-hand middle finger. Turn the dagger fingers around nine times leftwards and nine times rightwards, followed by "point respiration"

—exhale when pressing the fingers at the point and inhale when the fingers are lifted. Repeat three times altogether.

Detailed Movements

(1) Starting Form: when doing the Relaxed and Quiescent Sitting, place the hands flat on the upper parts of the thighs with the fingers together, palms facing each other at a slant (see Figure 67). When you calm down, raise the hands to *Dantian* and do the Three Deep Exhaling and Inhaling exercise (see Figure 68). The Three Exhaling and Inhaling Form in sitting position involves no crouching-and-standing-up movements. It requires only deep and long exhaling and inhaling. The rest of its method is the same as that of the Three Deep Exhaling and Inhaling in Standing Position. Its three open-and-close method is also the same as that of the Three Open-and-Close Form in Standing Position (see Figure 69).

(2) When you are through with the Starting Form, do

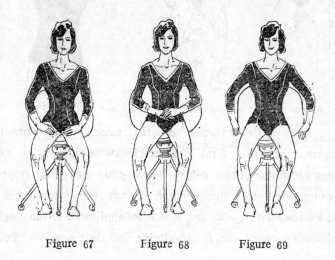

Figure 67   Figure 68   Figure 69

the *Yintang* Point Massage. Relax the wrists, bend the fingers slightly, drop the hands and move them up alongside the *Ren* Channel(the Midline of the body) (see Figure 70—71). When the hands reach the level of *Yintang*, both hands form "dagger fingers". Place the left-hand dagger finger on the *Yintang* Point, with, the right-hand dagger finger pressed at the point that separates the finger muscle and the nail of the middle finger of the left hand(see Figure 72). (Becuase if you press it completely on the nail, vital energy can not go through the nail, and if you press it on the finger muscle, the right-hand finger will slip off easily.)

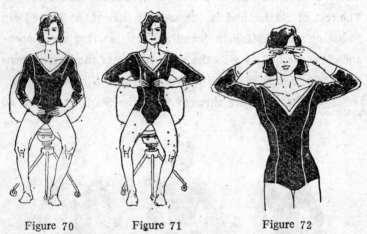

Figure 70　　　Figure 71　　　Figure 72

(3) Both fingers press on the same point. Turn the fingers nine times first counter-clockwise and then nine times clockwise. Press gently when you turn the fingers, avoid using force. This mehtod is not only applicable to the *Yintang* Point Massage, it is also applicable to the single-point massage of the *Fengfu* Point and the *Chengjiang* Point

and other points.

(4) "Point respiration" takes place when you gently press the *Yintang* Point after the turning of fingers. Exhale when pressing, and then, lift the fingers slightly (fingers slightly leave the point) and inhale. Repeat three times altogether.

(5) When the "point respiration" is over, move the hands down to *Dantian*.

2. *Baihui* and *Shuaigu* Point-Massage

Pithy Formula

The tops of the ears support the midlines of the wrists;
   the wrists are placed against the ears with *Zhongchong* touching the point.

The point that the fingertips touch is *Baihui*;
   once it is massaged, the head becomes clear.

The point facing *Laogong* is *Shuaigu*,
   which is used to treat cerebral trouble and headache.

Explanation

To decide the Point of *Baihui*, draw a straight line from each top of the ear to the top of the head. The point where the two lines meet is *Baihui*. If we place the midline of each wrist on top of the ear, the point where the two middle fingers meet is the *Baihui* Point. The *Shuaigu* Point is 1.5 *cun* inside the hairline above the ear, a little bit lower than the *Laogong* Point. But if the *Laogong* Point releases vital energy the *Shuaigu* Point could be stimulated. So this form of exercise involves two points. Massage the point in circles with palms, nine times forward and nine times backward, both palms and fingers moving. Then do "point respiration".

Those without high blood pressure or anal trouble need not do *Baihui* Point Massage.

Detailed Movements

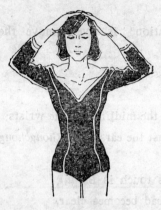
Figure 73

(1) Raise both hands, place the midline of the wrist, the root of the palm, on top of each ear. The two middle fingers meet at the *Baihui* Point. Do both the *Shuaigu* Point Massage and the *Baihui* Point Massage at the same time. For those who have hypotension do not massage *Baihui* with the middle fingers (see Figure 73).

(2) Massage the point with the palms in circles, nine times forward(massage the *Baihui* Point with the tips of the middle fingers simultaneously) and then nine times backward. Do "point respiration", pressing three times and breathing three times.

(3) Slip the palms backward to the back of the head.

3. *Fengfu* Point Massage

Pithy Formula

The *Fengfu* Point is inside the socket between the tendons of the neck. With dagger fingers you massage it in circles leftward and rightward. This massage can help keep the *Du* Channel uninterrupted.

158

Detailed Movements

(1) Do "point respiration" after applying massage to the *Fengfu* Point at the socket below the skull, nine times to the left and nine times to the right (see Figure 74). Restore the dagger fingers to normal position, and with the four fingers, stroke along the wandering nerve behind the ears to the front cheeks (see Figure 75).

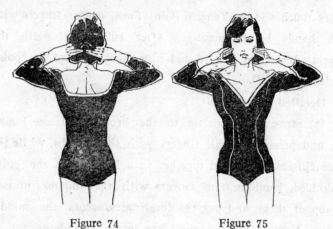

Figure 74   Figure 75

(2) When the fingers reach the lower part of the cheeks, move the hands down to *Dantian*.

4. *Yangbai* Point Massage

Pithy Formula

Bend the small finger and the thumb with
    the first three fingers extended.
Pay no attention to the position of the forefinger,
    but place the tip of the ring finger at the middle of
    each brow.
And the middle finger is right at the *Yangbai* Point.

159

With dagger fingers of both hands, you are ready for exercise.

Explanation

The *Yangbai* Point belongs to the Gallbladder Channel of Foot-Shaoyang. The method to decide this point is: With the first three fingers together, place the ring finger at the middle of the edge of each brow. The point that the middle finger touches is the *Yangbai* Point. Form dagger fingers with both hands before massage. After rubbing it with the fingers nine times inward and nine times outward, do "point respiration".

Detailed Movements

(1) Move the hands up to the brow level (see Figure 76), and press the small fingers with the thumbs, while the other fingers are joined together in a line. When the point is decided, bend the ring fingers with the thumbs pressed on top of them, and put the forefingers across the middle fingers. Now "dagger fingers" are formed(see Figure 77).

(2) Massage the *Yangbai* Point with dagger fingers of both hands, nine circles inwards and nine circles outwards. Then do "point respiration".

(3) Restore the dagger fingers of both hands to normal position, and move them to the top of the head. Then move them to the back of the head with fingers stroking the skin of the head. Now you are ready for the next movement— Tianzhu Massage.

5. *Tianzhu*(the celestial pillar) Massage

Pithy Formula

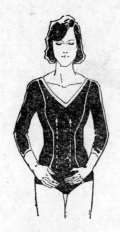
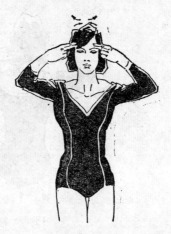

Figure 76   Figure 77

Tianzhu is a name given to the tendon at the back of
  the neck;
  it is not a point, nor is it fixed.
From top to bottom you knead six times;
  and six times of stroking is followed.

Explanation

Tianzhu refers to the main tendon at the back of the
neck, which plays a role similar to the *Tianzhu* point of
the Urinary Bladder Channel. Knead it six times before you
stroke it six times.

Detailed Movements

(1) Knead and nip the tendon at the back of the neck
with the thumbs and the first two fingers of both hands.
Start from the top, kneading and nipping six times downwards. This is called a round. Do 3—6 rounds (see Figure 78).
After this, stroke the main tendon from the top downwards

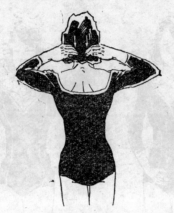

Figure 78

with all the fingers except the thumbs. Repeat 2 — 6 times.

(2) Stroke the neck with both hands from the back, under the cheeks, towards the front of the neck (i. e., along the wandering nerve), then move the hands down to *Dantian*.

6. *Touwei* Point Massage

Pithy Formula

The *Touwei* Point is at each of the temples.

 Apply massage to it with dagger fingers,

  turning both to the left and to the right,

  to relieve severe intermittent headache.

Explanation

The *Touwei* Point belongs to the Stomach Channel of Foot-*Yangming*, about 0.5 *cun* inside the hairline at the left and right temples. Massage the point with dagger fingers of both hands.

Detailed Movements

162

(1) Raise both hands up, and when they get near the hairline, move them to the temples. Massage the *Touwei* Point with dagger fingers of both hands(see Figure 79).

(2) Turn the fingers nine times inwards and nine times outwards before you do "point respiration".

(3) Restore the dagger fingers to normal position and

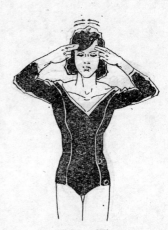

Figure 79

then move the hands to the back of the head with the fingers stroking the head skin. Form dagger fingers again and you are ready to massage the *Fengchi* Point.

7. *Fengchi* Point Massage

Pithy Formula

Massaging *Fengchi* can expel wind-evil,

with dagger fingers you massage the point.

Find the point by the side of the tendons at the back neck;

the point is at the same level of the ears.

Explanation

The *Fengchi* Point belongs to the Gallbladder Channel It is on the external side of the two tendons at the back of the neck at the same level of the ears. When you massage the point, there is a feeling of traction, and if you massage it with a little force, you have a sensation of radiation.

Detailed Movements

163

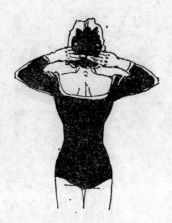

Figure 80

(1) Form dagger fingers with both hands. Massage the *Fengchi* Point in circles, first nine times inwards and then nine times outwards. After this, do "point respiration" (see Figure 80).

(2) Taking advantage of this position, pass both hands to the front neck under the cheeks with a stroking movement of the four fingers, and then lower both hands to *Dantian*.

8. *Taiyang* Point Massage

Pithy Formula

Taiyang is an Extraordinary point,

which has an extraordinary effect;

Massage it nine times forwards and nine times backwards, and

you will gain a satisfactory effect.

Explanation

Taiyang is an extra point, located in the fossa by the tip of the eyebrows. It is well-known that the point can be used to treat headaches. To apply massage to this point in term of *Qigong* will also produce a very good effect.

Detailed Movements

(1) Raise both hands to the level of the brows, stroke the brows with dagger fingers from the inner end to the outer

end and the *Taiyang* Point is
right in the fossa by the eyebrow (see Figure 81).

(2) Massage the *Taiyang*
Point in circles nine times
forward and nine times backward before you do "point
respiration".

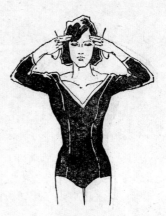

Figure 81

(3) After the massage, tap
the face with your fingers of
both hands onto the sides of
the cheeks and then move them down to *Dantian*. Go on to
the next method.

9. *Sizhukong* Point Massage

Pithy Formula

This point is close behind the brow tip,

where there is a small pit by the eye orbit.

With dagger fingers you massage the point nine times
back and forth, and

do the "point respiration" before you end the exercise.

Explanation

Sizhukong Point belongs to the Triple-Warmer Channel of
the Hand-*Shaoyang*. When pressing down the spot behind the
tip of the brow, you can feel a fossa resembling a gap
(further back is the *Taiyang* Point). This is ths *Sizhnkong*
Point.

Detailed Movements

165

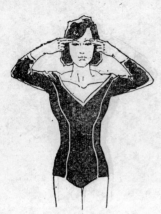

Figure 82

(1) Raise both hands to the level of the brows and form dagger fingers.

(2) Stroke the brows with the left and right dagger fingers from the inner ends to the outer ends. There is a small gap at the edge of the *Taiyang* Point. That is the *Sizhukong* Point (see Figure 82).

(3) Massage the point in circles, nine times forward and nine times backward before you do "point respiration".

(4) Tap the face with the tips of the four fingers of the two hands onto the cheeks and then move the hands down to *Dantian*.

10. Ear Formula

Pithy Formula

This massage involves two points.

You rub *Xiaguan* and *Tinggong* with your fingers.

The massage method is the same as the previous ones.

You can finish this massage at one run.

Explanation

The *Xiaguan* Point belongs to the Stomach Channel. It is at the joint between the ear and the jaw. You can spot the point by biting down the teeth and when you open your mouth, the point becomes flat. The *Tinggong* Point belongs to the Small Intestine Channel of *Taiyang*. It is at the front

166

part of the porusacusticus externus. Press it with the fingers with mouth shut, you will find it right at the back of the gums. Rub the two points at the same time.

Detailed Movements

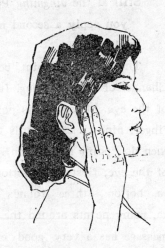

(1) After raising both hands to the level of *Yintang*, separate them. Move each hand along the exterior edge of the eyebrow to the tip of the brow. Then move it down to the front part of the ear. Bend the ring finger and the small finger. Place the thumb on top of the ring finger, the middle finger at the *Xiaguan* Point and the forefinger at the *Tinggong* Point (see Figure 83).

Figure 83

(2) Massage both points in circles at the same time, nine times forward and nine times backward before you do "point respiration". Then move both hands to *Dantian*.

11. Eye Massage

Pithy Formula

The small fingers tap at the *Jingming* Point,
      with all the other fingers bent in fists.
You massage the point nine times inwards and outwards, while
      breathing three times altogether.
Along the edge of the eye orbits,

you tap three times.

Once more you start from the eye corners,

and make three circles from the top.

Still at the *Jingming* Point,

you apply a second massage.

Explanation

The *Jingming* Point belongs to the Urinary Bladder Channel of Foot-*Taiyang*. It is located at the inner corner of the eye. Massage this point in circles with the small finger, nine times inwards and nine times outwards, and then do "point respiration". After this, tap along the orbit of the eye, first from bottom to the top and then from top to bottom, three rounds for each direction. In doing so, many points around the eye can be touched. So this massage has a very good effect in treating eye diseases, especially for glaucoma and contraction of visual field and other cases.

Detailed Movements

(1) Raise the hands to the level of the eyes.

(2) Put the thumb across the first three fingers and extend the small finger.

(3) Apply spot massage, with the small fingers, to the inner canthi, i. e., the *Jingming* Point, nine times inwards and nine times outwards. Then do "point respiration" (see Figure 84).

(4) Tap with the small fingers from the *Jingming* Point downward along the eye orbits through the outer canthi, the upper edge, and return to the *Jingming* point again. Do

three rounds altogether.

(5) Do the same for three rounds from the *Jingming* Point upwrads, through the upper edge, the outer canthi, the lower edge and return to the *Jingming* Point again (see Figure 85).

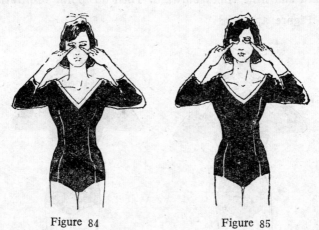

Figure 84   Figure 85

(6) Massage the *Jingming* Point again, nine times outward and nine times inward before doing "point respiration". Restore the hands to the normal positon and move the hands down to *Dantian*.

12. Nose Massage

Pithy Formula

Massage the nose before tapping the *Yingxiang* Point;
  you'll find the *Yingxiang* Point at about five *fen* beside the nose.

By massaging the *Yingxiang* point, you can treat colds;
  Yingxiang belongs to the Big Intestine Channel.

Detailed Movements

(1) Raise both hands to the level just below the eyes and form dagger fingers. Stroke the sides of the nose with dagger fingers up and down six times (see Figure 86).

(2) Massage the *Yingxiang* Point in circles nine times inward and nine times outward. Then do "point respiration" (see Figure 87).

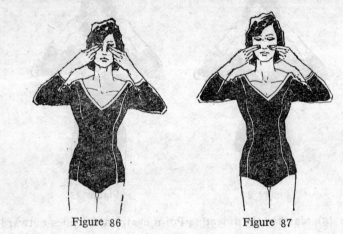

Figure 86   Figure 87

(3) Slip the dagger fingers down from the *Yingxiang* Point, by the outer corners of the mouth to the *Chengjiang* Point below the lower lip and now you are ready for the next massage.

13. *Chengjiang* Point Massage

Pithy Formula

The *Chengjiang* Point is below the lower lip,

in the very centre of which there is small pit.

You use dagger fingers to massage this Point.

Respiration makes the *Ren* Channel free from obstruction.

Explanation

170

The *Chengjiang* Point is a point of the *Ren* Channel. It is located right at the fossa below the lower lip. Massage the point in circles with dagger fingers nine times inward and nine times outward before doing "point respiration". The "point respiration" here can be longer so as to imagine the flowing of the vital energy through the *Ren* Channel and make the *Ren* Channel uninterrupted.

Detailed Movements

(1) Start from the preceding message. Press the left-hand dagger finger on the *Chengjiang* Point, and put the dagger finger of the right hand on the middle finger of the left hand (see Figure 88).

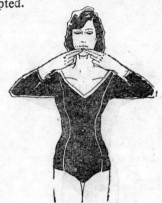

Figure 88

(2) Turn the fingers nine times inward and nine times outward before doing "point respiration".

(3) Restore the fingers to normal position before moving the hands down to *Dantian*.

14. Head-Massage Ending Form

Pithy Formula

Start from the hairline of the forehead, and
    with both plams you stroke the whole of the scalp.
When the hands reach the back of the neck,
    move them forward till under the cheeks.
After nine rounds of this ending form,

you'll feel satisfied and content.

Explanation

Stroke the top of the head to end the exercises. Though this step is very simple, yet it plays an important role. After doing it you'll feel comfortable with an effect of mental calmness and quiescence.

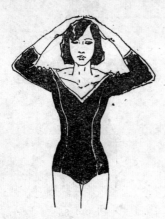
Figure 89

Detailed Movements

(1) Move both hands up to the hairline of the forehead and stroke the scalp from the front to the back. When the hands reach the back of the neck, move them to the front under the cheeks along the wandering nerve. Lower the hands to *Dantian*. Repeat nine times altogether (see Figure 89).

(2) Do the Three Open-and-Close Form and the Three Deep Exhaling and Inhaling Form when the hands get to *Dantian* after the ninth time.

(3) After the Three Deep Exhaling and Inhaling exercise, put both hands on the thighs, ready for the Relaxed and Quiescent exercise in sitting position.

The method of Relaxed and Quiescent Sitting exercise is quite simple, yet as far as basic *Qigong* technique is concerned, it is the main method of the quiescent exercises.

(4) When doing the quiescent sitting breathing, beginners can adopt the natural breathing method, but it can be

replaced with the abdominal breathing method after some practice(say, three months). There are two different ways of abdominal respiration. One is called "normal abdominal respiration" which involves swelling up the abdomen when inhaling and contracting the abdomen when exhaling. The other is called "paradoxical respiration" which involves swelling the abdomen when exhaling and contracting the abdomen when inhaling. Both methods can be adopted.

(5) The length of time for sitting varies. Tranquility can be gained within ten minutes.

(6) Quiescent Sitting can be performed immediately after the Head-Massaging and Mind-Tranquilizing Pattern. It can also be performed independently.

IV. Kidney-Massaging and Essence-Benefiting Pattern
Pithy Formula
At your bedside you can do the Starting Form,
massage the *Shenshu* Point till it is warm.
The hand presses *Shenhu* and turns gently,
24 times inward and 24 times outward.
Do "point respiration" three times;
do not look when your eyelids have dropped.
The left hand gently massages the *Yongquan* Point,
first a hundred times clockwise and then counterclockwise.
"Point respiration" should not be forgotten.
Massage the point as slowly as hypnotizing;
point facing point is the key point.
Put the right-hand *Laogong* Point over *Dantian*;

do not neglect "point respiration" while pressing.

Rub the left foot after rubbing the right;

the method is the same but the direction is opposite.

As this massage has a long history,

it can invigorate vital energy.

Explanation

This *Qigong* pattern is simple and easy to perform. It is most appropriate to practise at night before bedtime. when doing it before bedtime, the performers, very often, fall asleep without finishing it. This method is most effective to treat insomnia. A few people, however, get excited when doing this exercise. If this happens, you can either do the *Shenshu* Point Massage alone, or do the *Yongquan* Point massage alone. You can also do both at an earlier hour, e. g. 17—19 o'clock. In short, one can decide according to his own constitution(This pattern requires the eyes to be shut slightly).

This pattern involves two parts: the *Shenshu* Point Massage and the *Yongquan* Point Massage. The *Shenshu* Point is below the spinous process of the second lumbar vertebra about 1.5 *cun* aside. The *Yongquan* Point is at the centre of the arch of the foot. Bend the five toes of your foot, you'll find the point at the fossa in the front of the foot arch. It is required that the middle finger should be placed right at the *Shenshu* Point when you perform. Turn the hands 24 times clockwise and 24 times counter-clockwise(inwards and out-wards). (Keep the hands to the point and avoid using effort.) Massage the *Yongquan* Point with the *Laogong* Point facing

174

it, 100 times clockwise and 100 times counter-clockwise.

Detailed Movements

(1) Before going to bed, dismiss all distracting thoughts. when you are free from worries and calmed down, do the Relaxed and Quiescent Standing, the Three Deep Exhaling and Inhaling, and the Starting Form of the Three Open-and-Close in front of your bed. You can also do the Three Deep Exhaling and Inhaling, and the Starting Form of the Three Open-and-Close in sitting positon.

(2) Move both hands to the *Shenshu* Point along the waist. After a dozen times of massaging up and down, the back waist will get warm. Then, press the two *Zhongchong* Points of both middle fingers on the left and right *Shenshu* points separately. (Those who are comparatively fat and have difficulty in performing this way, can press the outer *Laogong* Point on the *Shenshu* Point.) Turn both hands 24 times inwards and 24 times outwards. "To turn inward" means the fingertips of both hands move towards the centre of the waist, while "to turn outward" suggests the fingertips of both hands turn apart outwards from the centre of the waist. Keep the hands on the *Shenshu* Point when turning them round so as to make the skin and muscles turn slightly.

(3) After 24 times of inward massage and 24 times outward massage, do "point respiration" three times. Exhale when the palms pressing gently, and inhale when the palms lifted(see Figure 90—91).

(4) Move both hands back to the Middle *Dantian* along

175

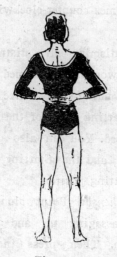

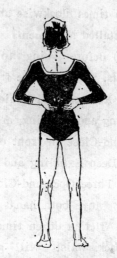

Figure 90   Figure 91

the waist before doing the Three Open-and-Close Form, then repeat the massage of the *Shenshu* Point three times.

(5) After doing the *Shenshu* Point Massage three times, do the Three Open-and-Close and the Three Deep Exhaling and Inhaling once more before you start the next massage—The *Yongquan* Point Massage.

(6) Sitting on the bed, turn the body to the right and lift the right leg and foot on the bed with the left foot hanging from the edge of the bed.

(7) With the right hand on *Dantian* (or on the *Shenshu* Point), put the left hand on the *Yongquan* Point of the right foot with the *Laogong* Point facing it(see Figure 92—93).

(8) Turn the left hand round without leaving the point. After 100 times of counter-clockwise massage, do

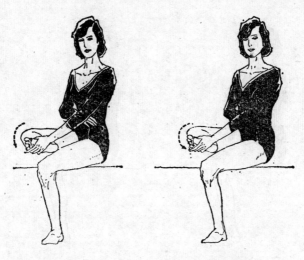

Figure 92   Figure 93

"point respiration". Then turn the hand clockwise 100 times before doing "point respiration" again. When massaging *Yongquan*, hold the right hand still on *Dantian* (or on *Shenshu*), but while doing "point respiration", press it when exhaling and lift it up when inhaling.

(9) When doing the Three Open-and-Close in sitting position, hold the left leg and foot bent on the bed, the right foot hanging straight from the bed edge.

(10) Put the left hand at *Dantian* or *Shenshu*, and start to massage the *Yongquan* Point with the right hand using the same method as explained previously(see Figure 94,95).

(11) After the left-foot *Yongquan* Point Massage, do the Three Open-and-Close in sitting position and the Three Deep Exhaling and Inhaling (in sitting position) to end the exercise. After sitting quiescently for a while, gotosleep.

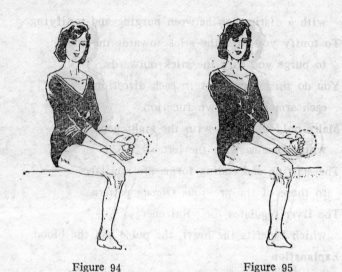

|Figure 94|Figure 95|

(12) The vital energy will be easily dispersed if it is not brought back to *Dantian*. So be sure to end the exercise after practising. If you suffer from insomnia and you feel sleepy after the *Yongquan* Point massage, you can go to bed without doing the ending form. Do not do the ending form until you are recovered from insomnia.

Ⅴ. **The Relaxed and Quiesccent *Qi*-Regulating Pattern**
 Pithy Formula
 The stick which you grip in your hand,
  is less than a *chi* in length.
 The exercise has a long history, and
  its technique is similar to *Taiji*.
 With palms rotating the ends of the stick,
  you rub the *Laogong* Point to dredge the channels.
 The exercise emphasizes quiescence and relaxation,

with a distinction between purging and tonifying.
To tonify you turn the stick towards the body,
  to purge you turn the stick outwards.
You do this four times in each direction,
  each arm has its own function.
Males hold the stick with the right hand,
  while females with the left.
The starting and ending forms are similar,
  to those of the previous Qigong patterns.
The liver regulates the vital energy,
  which benefits the heart, the pulse and the blood.

Explanation

The Relaxed and Quiescent Qi-Regulating Pattern is an exercise with instrument, so it is also called "Small Stick Exercise". Prepare a stick which is about 8—9 cun in length, and is thick enough so that the thumb and the middle finger can easily grasp. Both ends of the stick should be round and smooth so that the palms can rub them easily. It is most desirable to have the stick made of a piece of wood from a Chinese prickly ash tree, though other wood can also serve the purpose.

This exercise has the effect of dispersing the depressed liver-energy and invigorate the tendons. It also helps to dredge the channels and collaterals, and to promote smooth circulation of blood and vital energy and to tranquilize the mind. It can rectify deviations of Qigong exercises through practice. That is why it is called the Relaxed and Quiescent Qi-Regulating Pattern. This exercise has a very good tonifying and purging effect. When doing the exercise, "to turn the stick away from the body" means "to purge", while "to turn the stick towards the body" means "to tonify". The performer can decide the direction according to his own condition. The theory is the same as the tonifying and purging principles of acupuncture. The purging method suits sthenia-syndromes and the tonifying method suits the asthenia-syndromes. When the patient's condition improves, normal tonifying and purging methods will be adopted.

1. Crouching Form

Pithy Formula

With both hands rotating the stick near *Dantian*,

have the legs bent, the body dropped but kept straight.

Keep the hips as if sitting and the spine as if standing,

the waist is relaxed and the vital energy is flowing.

Explanation

After the starting form, hold the stick between the palms, and rotate it in front of *Dantian*. While crouching, keep the stick rotating and hold the upper part of the body straight, the seat slightly dropped and the spine erect, avoiding stiffness in the waist. In the course of rising and crouching, the sacral bone is loosened and you will feel that the vital energy is pouring into the *Yongquan* Point. Do this pattern four times.

Detailed Movements

(1) The starting form of the Relaxed and Quiescent

Qi-Regulating Pattern also involves the relaxed and quiescent standing (see Figure 96), the three deep exhaling and inhaling and the three open-and-close (see Figure 97). But when

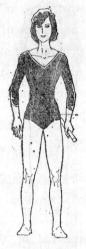

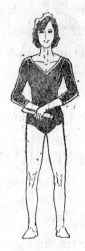

Figure 96   Figure 97

doing the starting form of this pattern, you perform with a stick in your right hand (females, with a stick in the left hand). When doing the three deep exhaling and inhaling you put the left hand (females, the right hand) at *Dantian* and hold the stick with the right hand (females, with the left hand), and rest the spot where the thumb and the middle finger meet on top of the outer *Laogong* Point of the left hand (the right hand of a female). The other movements of the three deep exhaling and inhaling are the same as those of the exercise without the stick, which are omitted here. The method to do the three open-and-close is also the same except the stick held in the hand (see **Figure**

98.99).

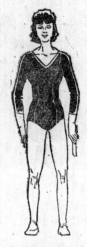 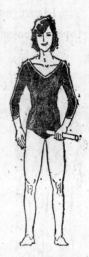

Figure 98   Figure 99

(2) After the starting form, put one end of the stick on the *Laogong* Point of the left palm (right palm for females) and the other end of the stick on the *Laogong* Point of the right palm. Rotate the stick with the right hand supported by the left hand. Rotate it with the left hand, supported by the right hand. Rotate the stick only with the palm center, avoiding using fingers. Hold both hands at the same level while rotating (see Figure 100).

(3) When crouching, do not exert yourself. Those who are weak or have trouble in the lower limbs can crouch slightly. Those who have better health conditions can crouch to the extent that the thighs are flat (see Figure 101). Be sure to crouch as if riding a horse with the knees in the front and the feet in parallel, avoiding sticking out the seat

(see Figure 102).

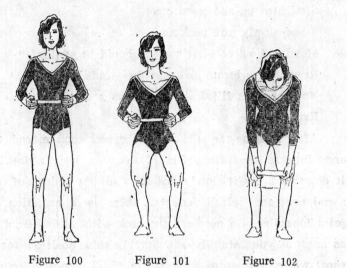

Figure 100   Figure 101   Figure 102

(4) Thoughts are concentrated on the tip of the sacral bone. Keep the head suspended, so that the head and the sacral bone are in a line, the spine erect, and the waist extended——to have the head suspended and the sacral bone dropped, the joints of the bones must be loosened.

(5) After this, do the three deep exhaling and inhaling and the three open-and-close. Get ready for the next exercise.

2. Back-Bending Form

Pithy Formula

Rotate the stick and bend the back
    as if to draw a bow.

Every joint of the spinal vertebra should be loosened.

Stretch the arms and suspend the head

as if to have it weighed.

Straighten up and stand erect

and slowly you perform.

Massive flow of vital energy should be avoided.

Regulate the breath and ease the mind

Your heart is filled with calmness and peace.

Explanation

After rotating the stick, bend the back and extend the arms forward, head dropped as if there is weight drawing it downward. Do it slowly and relax all the joints of the sacral bone and spinal vertebra. There is a sensation of joint loosening. Do not bend the back with strain. Bend it as much as you naturally can. Stay in this position for a short while. The words at heart are "Stop dropping. Restore to the original position". When straightening up and restoring to the original position. There is still a sensation of loosening in the sacral bone and spinal vertebra. Avoid impatience when practising. Impatience causes the vital energy to surge up. The key point in bending the back is to have "tranquil heart-energy and natural relaxation".

Do this form four times.

Detailed Movements

(1) Keep the stick rotating incessantly when bending the back, with the knees slightly bent, avoiding straightness. Loosen the joints one by one.

(2) When dropping the head, keep the head, the neck and the spine in a line. Do not drop the head too low or it will cause the vital energy to surge up.

(3) The extent of back-bending depends on the individual's condition. Any strain should be avoided. For some people the hands may reach the ground, while for others, it will be fine for the hands to fall below the knees. Do not drop the head too much when bending the back or it will cause dizziness (see Figure 103). Patients of hypertension must bear the key rules in mind, not to perform too fast.

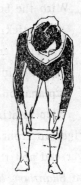

Figure 103

The mind should be calm and the breath should be steady.

(4) When straightening up and restoring to the original position, let every joint of the spinal vertebra loosen.

(5) Do the three deep exhaling and inhaling and the three open-and-close. Move on to the next form.

3. Back-Relaxing Form

Pithy Formula

To relax the waist, the stick is held upright,
  with lower end at *Shanzhong* and upper at *Yintang.*
Step out with the left foot at the same time, and
  raise the stick to the left supported by the right hand.
With the stick reaching the right ear, the body leans
  back, and the stick rotates and hides itself behind the head.
The right hand is up and the left is down,

you rotate the stick and move it to the left ear.
With the body restored to the upright position,
     the stick rotates in front of your body.
The vital energy guides you through the exercise, and
     your joints are loosened and your tendons relaxed.

Explanation

After rotating the stick in front of *Dantian*, hold it upright in front of the chest, with the right hand at its lower end and the left hand at its upper end. Keep it upright with *Shanzhong* as the limit of its lower end, and *Yintang* as the limit of its upper end. Turn the waist leftwards with both hands holding the stick. When the stick reaches the side of the left ear, keep it turning. Move both hands upwards and backwards. The body slightly leans back. The stick may be held at the level of *Fengfu*. Relax the waist. Keep rotating the stick. Turn the lumbar region to the left with the left hand at the lower end of the stick and the right hand at the upper end till the stick reaches the side of the left ear. Restore the waist to the upright position. Rotate the stick with both hands and move it to the front of the chest. Move the upright stick back to the front of *Dantian* and rotate it with both hands at the same level. Do 4 times. Then step out with the right foot. With the left hand at the upper end of the stick, rotate it to the left. Relax the waist and lean back. Repeat another four times in the same way as mentioned above, but in the opposite direction.

Detailed Movements

(1) Rotate the stick with both hands in front of *Dantian*. Step out with the left foot. Place the stick upright between *Shanzhong* and *Yintang* with the left hand at the upper end and the right hand supporting the lower end (see Figure 104).

(2) Turn the waist to the right. Keep rotating the stick with both hands and move it to the front of the right ear (see Figure 105).

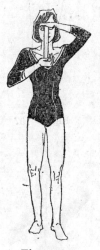
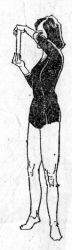

Figure 104   Figure 105

(3) Relax the waist and lean back slightly. Move the stick over head with the left hand and rotate it at the *Fengfu* point behind the head, both hands at the same level (see Figure 106,107).

(4) Move the left hand down and the right hand up and the stick moves to the front of the left ear.

(5) Rotate the stick with both palms and move it to the

187

front of the body (see Figure 108)

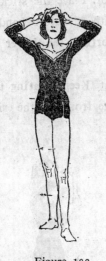
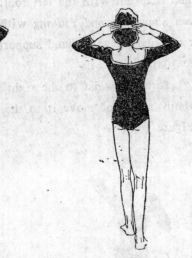

Figure 106   Figure 107

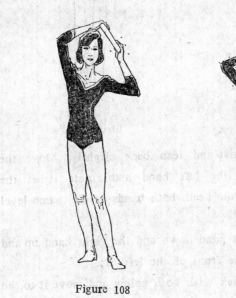
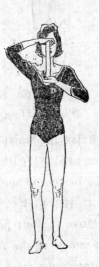

Figure 108   Figure 109

(6) Repeat four times. After the three open-and-close exercise, step out with the right foot. Set the stick upright and turn it leftwards with the right hand at the upper end and the left hand at the lower end. Turn to the left (see Figure 109). Do another four times in the same way mentioned above, but in the opposite direction.

(7) After the three open-and-close and the three deep exhaling and inhaling, do the next pattern.

4. Arm-Revolving and Waist-Turning Form

Pithy Formula

The empty hand takes the lead,

the stick follows but in the opposite direction.

The left hand moves past the *Jianjing* Point, and

then falls down after rising above *Baihui*.

The right hand moves past the *Qimen* Point, and

then falls down after rising over the head.

If the stick causes disturbance when passing over *Baihui*,

let it pass over any other place to avoid dizziness.

Explanation

To do this form, the empty hand goes ahead. Step out with the left foot. Hold the stick with the right hand. The left hand moves up to the shoulder along the right side of the body, and then moves down after it rises above *Jianjing* and *Baihui*. The right hand that holds the stick starts to move when the left hand rises over head and rises, from the right to the left, via the *Qimen* Point on the left side above the shoulder and over the *Baihui* Point on top of the head.

It then moves down along the right side. When the empty hand moves, from the left, rightwards and then upwards, hold the right foot weightless and the waist turns with the hand rightwards, leftwards and rightwards. The hand that holds the stick moves from the left to the right. When the empty hand goes up, hold the left foot weightless. The waist turns rightwards, backwards and leftwards. Do the ending form, the three open-and-close, the three deep exhaling and inhaling and the relaxed and quiescent standing. This is for males. For females, the direction is just the opposite.

Detailed Movements (Take the females for example)

(1) Hold the stick in the left hand (in the right hand for a male) and do the relaxed and quiescent standing.

(2) Step out with the right foot. The right hand moves up from the left side of the lower abdomen along the left side of the body, via the *Qimen* Point on the left side to the shoulder, rising over the *Jianjing* Point and the *Baihui* Point (see Figure 110) and moves down natually along the right side.

(3) When the right hand reaches the *Baihui* Point, the left hand, holding the stick, turns with the waist and moves to the right side of the lower abdomen. Then it immediately rises up after passing by *Qimen* and rises above *Baihui*. Then it falls down naturally along the left side (see Figure 111).

If you have disturbances such as dizziness when the stick passes over *Baihui*, you may let it pass over *Congmen* or the front part of the top.

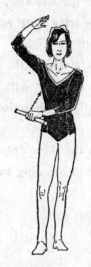
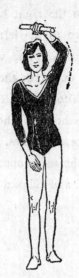

Figure 110

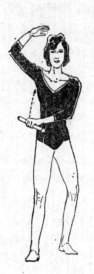
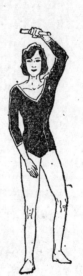

Figure 111

(4) When the right hand reaches the left side, the head and waist turn to the left. When the left hand reaches the right side, the head and waist turn to the right.

(5) Step out with the right foot and turn the waist. Do four times altogether. Then, step forward with the left foot. The method is the same but the direction is the opposite. Repeat 4 times.

(6) Do the three open-and-close, the three deep exhaling and inhaling, and relaxed and quiescent standing to end the exercise.

Book III

CONTINUATION
OF *QIGONG* PATTERNS

Chapter 1
Cancer-Treating *Qigong* Patterns

I. **A Contrast Between Cancer-Treating *Qigong* Patterns and the Five Basic *Qigong* patterns**

Cancer-treating *Qigong* Patterns are some special *Qigong* patterns based on the five basic *Qigong* patterns mentioned before. The design of these patterns lays stress on treating the sthenia-syndrome by purgation. The following is a comparison between the cancer-treating *Qigong* patterns, their starting forms and the five basic *Qigong* patterns.

1. Starting Forms

(1) The Relaxed and Quiescent Form in Standing Position: When used to treat cancer, the performance of this starting form is the same as that of the five basic *Qigong* patterns.

(2) The Three Deep Exhaling and Inhaling Form: When used to treat cancer, this starting form is changed into the Three Deep Inhaling and Exhaling Form. That is to inhale first and then exhale deeply. When the two hands are overlapped, inhale through the nose in standing position. Then crouch and exhale deeply through the nose at the same time. Stand up after the deep exhaling. Repeat three times.

(3) The Three Open-and-Close Form: To treat cancer, this starting form is the same as that of the five basic Qigong patterns.

2. The Breath-Regulating and Qi-Reenforcing Pattern

(1) The Rudimentary Method to Strengthen Health: When used to treat cancer, the performance of this method is the same.

(2) The Fixed-Step Blowing Method: For the treatment of cancer, the performance of this method is to step out with the left foot first and then the right foot, with the heel touching the ground and the big toe not touching the ground. The remainder of the method is the same as the five basic Qigong patterns.

(3) The Blowing Method to Strengthen the kidney: For the treatment of cancer, the performance of this method is the same as the five basic Qigong patterns except that this method lays stress on tonification and the performer should step out with the right foot first.

(4) The Blowing Method to Strengthen the Lung, the Spleen and the Kidney: To treat cancer, the performance of this method is to step out with the left foot first, and the remainder of the method is the same as the five basic Qigong patterns.

(5) The Blowing Method to Strengthen the Heart: To treat cancer, the performance of this method is the same as the five Qigong patterns.

3. The Toe-Raised Transport and Conversion Pattern

(1) The Open-and-Close Method at the Three Dantians:

196

For the treatment of cancer, the Deep Breathing Open-and-Close Method is adopted.

(2) The Toe-Raised Slow Walking Method: It is inadvisable for cancer patients to perform this *Qigong* exercise before they are fully recovered from the disease. To do this exercise, the performer starts from the preceding position with the right foot in the front and steps out with the left foot first. Perform the "nine-step *daoyin*" twice.

(3) The Open-and-Close Method at the Two Ɔantians: Step out with the left foot first. The rest is the same as the five basic patterns.

(4) Abdomen-Kneading: The performance of this exercise is the same as before. But when patients who suffer from intestinal and gastric cancer use this method, they should not exercise too much mental control.

4. The Head-Massaging and Mind-Tranquilizing Pattern

The performance of this pattern is the same as that of the Head-Massaging and Mind-Tranquilizing Pattern of the five basic patterns mentioned before.

5. The Kidney-Massaging and Essence-Benefiting Pattern

The performance of this pattern is the same as that of the Kidney-Massaging and Essence-Benefiting Pattern of the five basic patterns mentioned before.

6. The Relaxed and Quiescent *Qi*-Regulating Pattern

The performance of this pattern is basically the same as that of the Relaxed and Quiescent *Qi*-Regulating Pattern mentioned before. The only difference is to step out with the right foot in this pattern wherever to step out with the left foot in the former pattern.

Ⅱ. Three Special Cancer-Treating *Qigong* Methods

1. The Blowing and Fast Walking Method

The Blowing and Fast Walking Method is a supplementary *Qigong* exercise to the Breath-Regulating and *Qi*-Reenforcing Pattern. The Blowing and Fast Walking Method is based on the Blowing Method to Strengthen the Kidney and can be classified into three kinds according to the different walking speeds:

(1) The Fast Blowing Method: Step out with the left foot first and breathe in through the nose at the same time. Then, step out with the right foot and breathe out through the nose to form an even breathing of air-expulsion with inhaling for one step followed by exhaling for another step. The two hands swing naturally with the walking pace. The method is the same as the Blowing Method to Strengthen the Kidney. The key point is that the head leads the waist in turning and the arms swing with the waist to make the steps. Make 70-100 steps per minute.

(2) The Moderate Blowing Method: Breathe in and out while stepping out with the left foot, and then step out with the right foot while breathing in and out through the nose. Keep on walking with one step accompanying one respiration.

This method is mainly applied to early-stage cancer cases and is especially suitable for patients of gastric and intestinal cancer.

(3) The Slow Blowing Method: Step out with the left foot first and then with the right foot. Every step is

accompanied by two inhalings and one exhaling. That is, touch the ground with the heel while taking two inhalings and then touch the ground with the front part of the sole while taking one exhaling. Since one step involves three breathing movements, the walking speed should be a bit slower, appropriately 60 steps a minute.

2. The Deep Breathing Open-and-Close Method

This method is the Open-and-Close Method at the Three *Dantians* supplemented by deep inhaling and exhaling. The breathing *daoyin* of this method requires inhaling through the nose and exhaling through the mouth and exhaling after inhaling. Both inhaling and exhaling should be gentle, thin, even, long and slow. On the basis of opening and closing at the three *Dantians*, perform again the open-and-close at the Upper *Dantian* and Middle *Dantian* supplemented by three times of deep inahling and exhaling. That is, perform four times of open-and-close at the Upper *Dantian* and Middle *Dantian*. The details are as follows:

Deep Inhaling and Exhaling at the Upper *Dantian*: For the first open-and-close, do not exhale: only inhale when closing. For the second open-and-close, exhale when opening, and inhale when closing. For the third open-and-close, exhale when opening, and inhale when closing. When performing the fourth open-and-close, exhale when opening, and breathe naturally when closing. To perform the open-and-close at the Middle *Dantian*, the inhaling and exhaling method is the same as that at the Upper *Dantian*. The open-and-close at the Lower *Dantian* is not accompanied by deep exhaling and inhaling (natural breathing). Step out with the left foot first and turn the body round in the direction as the sun goes, for the first four times, and then step out with the right foot and turn the body round counter to the direction of the sun's movment for the second four times.

The Deep Breathing Open-and-Close Method is the Open-and-Close Method at the Three *Dantians* of the Toe-Raised Transport and Conversion Pattern in which the "tonification method" has been replaced by the "purgation method". This is aimed to treat the sthenia-syndrome by purgation, to remove blood stasis and to disperse stagnation. Its function is to dredge the channels and collaterals and promote the internal energy for the rising of *yang* and the falling of *yin*. Calming the *yin* and suppressing the *yang* can promote the flowing of vital energy and blood through the five solid organs and six hollow organs, and has the effect of eliminating the evil factors and supporting the healthy energy. The main points of this method are as follows:

(1) The exhaling and inhaling should be gentle, thin, even and long; and the mind should not concentrate on the expansion of the lung region. Do not use the normal abdominal breathing. Focus the mind on the general breathing Inhale and exhale as if through every pore on the body surface.

(2) When breathing, be sure to have the whole body relaxed. The key point to relax the whole body is to relax the waist. The performer will have a sensation of relaxation

and happiness when exhaling, inhaling, opening and closing with the whole body, especially the waist, relaxed.

3. The Aspirating and Word-Pronouncing Method

This is a sound-uttering method to relax the throat by letting air pass through it. This method involves a series of word-pronouncing exercises. The performer starts from the low-pitch sound of *"duo"*, trying to experience the characteristics of pronouncing with a relaxed vocal cord, and then gradually works up to sounds of higher pitch.

The pronunciations of the sounds must be correct; the resonant effects of the sounds must be brought into full play and thus the sound waves will be transmitted to the lesion spots of the internal organs. So resonance is produced and good results are effected.

A moderate volume of sound is considered as the standard for pronunciation. With low-volume pronunciation, the performer can easily feel where the sound waves reach and acquire resonant effect, but the amplitude of the sound wave is not wide enough and its vibrational force is very weak. On the other hand, high-volume pronunciation is liable to create tension and can cause mistakes. The said moderate volume is decided by the individual's own voice. It should be limited to the range in which the performer's voice does not strain and the performer can raise or lower his voice effortlessly. The volume of sound uttered also depends on the performer's health condition. People who are physically weak can mainly take the Breath-Regulating and Qi-Reenforcing Pattern and do not practise the word-pronouncing method until they feel energetic. To practise the word-pronouncing method, the performer should start from the low-volume and increase it gradually. Diseases of different parts of the body require different volumes. For example, patients with heart or lung trouble can preferably take the low and moderate volume pronunciation; patients with liver, spleen and stomach diseases can take the moderate- and high-volume pronunciation and patients with kidney and intestinal diseases can use the moderate- and high-volume pronunciation.

According to the relationship between the five pronunciations and the five solid organs recorded in *Nei Jing*, the pronouncing method is as follows: "*Gong*——the sound of the spleen; *shang*——the sound of the kidney; *guo*——the sound of the liver; *zheng*——the sound of the heart; *yu*——the sound of the kidney." Every sound is further classified into two sounds—a high-pitched sound and a low-pitched sound. The high-pitched sound is pronounced in the first tone and the low-pitched sound is pronounced in the third tone. The relationship between the five pronunciations and the five solid organs as well as the number of pronunciations are listed in the following table:

Like other methods, the starting form should be performed and the performer should get relaxed as much as possible before pronouncing the sounds. After the starting form, put the hands on the back and press the middle finger with the thumb at the *Shenshu* Point and then pronounce the sounds. Pronounce the high-pitched sound first with the head slightly dropped and the body turning from

Table 6

		Wood	fire	earth	gold	water
pronunciation	high-pitched, first tone	guō	zhēng	gōng	shāng	yū
	low-pitched, third tone	guǒ	zhěng	gōng	shāng	yǔ
range of treatment	solid organs	liver	heart	spleen	lung	kidney
	hollow organs	gallbladder	small intestine	stomach	large intestine	urinary bladder
treatment	the body	tendon	pulse	muscle	skin	bone
	the orifices	eye	tongue	mouth	nose	ear
number of pronunciations		8	7	10	9	6

left to right. When the lingering sound ends and the body resumes its normal position, breathe in the fresh air and breathe out the carbon dioxide through the nose. Then, regulate the breath naturally. Pronounce the low-pitched sound when the breath is normal and the heart is calmed down. The method of pronouncing the low-pitched sound is the same as that of pronouncing the high-pitched sound except that the body turns from right to left. After pronouncing the high-pitched and low-pitched sounds, perform the open-and-close once. This is one round. When the number of pronunciations are performed according to the requirements, by the different solid and hollow organs, the exercise can be ended by performing the Three Open-and-Close Form and the Three Deep Exhaling and Inhaling Form.

As a beginner, the performer should not be anxious to complete the required number of pronunciations. He can divide it into several parts and pronounce a different number of sounds at a different stage and gradually reach the required number. So the performer can adapt himself to the method and not get tired. For example, the sound "shang" is pronounced nine times for each exercise in the case of a lung disease. But a beginner may pronounce it three times and gradually work up to six times in twenty days. Then, in another thirty days he can reach the required number of times.

The choice of sound must suit the specific disease. Usually the "zheng" sound is pronounced for patients with heart trouble, the "shang" sound for patients with lung trouble, the "guo" sound for patients with liver diseases, the "gong" sound for patients with spleen diseases and the "yu" sound for patients with kidney diseases. Patients with cancer should mainly pronounce the "purgation sound" "ha". The "ha" is pronounced nine times. Its high-pitched sound is "hā", in the first tone and its low-pitched sound is "hǎ", in the third tone. After pronouncing the sound "ha" for a certain period of time, add the specific sounds for specific internal organs in the light of different diseases. That is, add "shang" for a patient with lung cancer and "guo" for a patient with liver cancer.

Patients of cancer should pronounce "xi" when their blood picture is low after chemotherapy. The sound "xi" is pronounced six times. Its high-pitched sound is "xi", in the first tone and its low-pitched sound is "xi" in the third tone. This sound is dropped and replaced by the sound "ha" or the sound for the specific internal organ as soon as the blood picture becomes normal.

Patients with stomach cancer should not pronounce the sound "gong", the specific sound for stomach. Instead, the "dong" sound should be pronounced. The "dong" sound is pronounced ten times. Its high-pitched sound is "dōng", in the first tone and its low-pitched sound is "dǒng", in the third tone.

Patients with benign tumour and brain cancer should pronounce the sound "duo". The "duo" sound is pronounced ten times. Its high-pitched sound is "duō" in the first tone and its low-pitched sound is *"duǒ"*, in the third tone.

See Figures 112—119 for the word-pronouncing method to treat cancer.

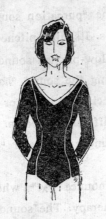 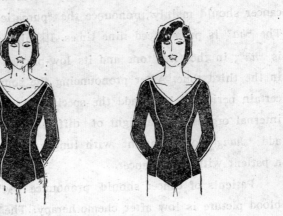

Figure 112 (duo) Figure 113 (ha)

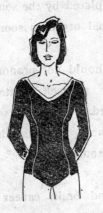 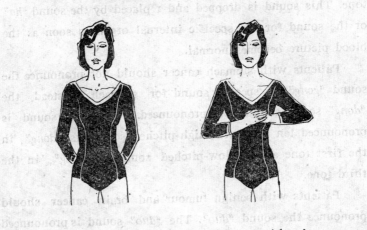

Figure 114 (xi) Figure 115 (zheng)

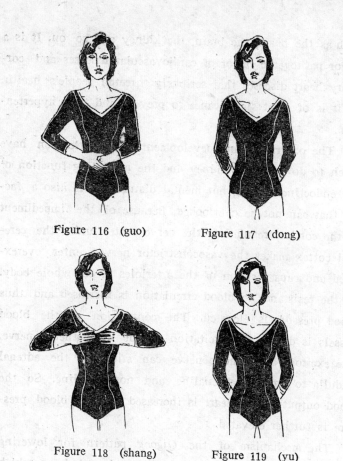

Figure 116 (guo) Figure 117 (dong)

Figure 118 (shang) Figure 119 (yu)

Chapter 2
The Hypertension–Treating Pattern

Hypertension is one of the common diseases in China.
It can cause a series of other diseases to the main organs

such as the heart, the brain, the kidney and so on. It is a major pathogenic factor of cardiovascular diseases and coronary heart diseases that seriously threaten people's health. So it is of great significance to prevent and treat hypertension.

The occurrence and development of hypertension have much to do with the kidney and the regulating function of the endocrine system, but mental disturbance is also a factor that can not be overlooked. Because of the impediment of the cortical regulation, the nerve center under the cerebral cortex makes the vasoconstrictor nerve center overexcited and causes spasm of the arterioles of the whole body. So the resistance to blood circulation is increased and thus blood pressure is elevated. The contraction of the blood vessels is due to the excitation of the sympathetic nerve. The excitory sympathetic nerve can stimulate the adrenal medulla to produce adrenaline and noradrenaline. So the blood output of the heart is increased and the blood pressure is further elevated.

The mechanism of the *Qigong* pattern for lowering blood pressure depends on relaxation and naturalness, which can put the cerebral cortex into an inhibitory and resting state. So this *Qigong* pattern has the function of healing trauma and adjusting imbalances. During the *Qigong* exercises, the gentle, thin, even and long exhalings and inhalings may excite the parasympathetic nerve. So the peripheral blood vessels will dilate and the resistance to blood circulation will be reduced, thus producing a blood pressure-lowering effect. The following is an introduction to the detailed performance of the Hypertension-Treating *Qigong* Pattern.

Ⅰ. *Baihui* Point Massage

1. Starting Form: The method is the same as what was explained before.

2. Hand-Over-Head Method: Lift both hands from the Middle *Dantian* along the *Chong* Channel with palms facing the belly. Lift them with the fingertips downward till the top of the head and then turn the downward fingertips of both hands to point at each other. Both hands cover the top of the head without touching it. Keep the hands at about 15 cm away from the top of the head for 2-3 minutes, and then lower them to massage the *Baihui* Point with the palms (see Figures 120—121).

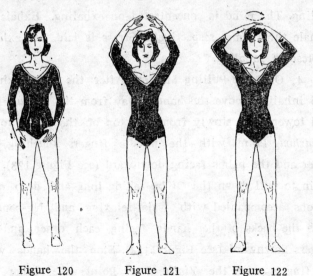

Figure 120   Figure 121   Figure 122

3. *Baihui* Point Massage: place the left hand (the right hand for the female) on the *Baihui* Point, and the right hand (the left hand for the female) on top of the left hand (the right hand for the female). Massage the *Baihui* Point with the inner *Laogong* Point of the upper hand resting at the outer *Laogong* Point of the lower hand. Turn gently twelve times in the order of left, front, right, back and left, and then twelve times again in the order of right, front, left, and back. (see Figure 122) (The order is just the opposite for the female, i.e., first back, left, front, right, and then left, back, right, front, left.) After this, exhale deeply with both hands massaging the *Baihui* Point gently. Crouch a little when exhaling. After exhaling, both hands move a little away from the *Baihui* Point and inhale. Do not stand up when inhaling. Stand up only after inhaling. The mind is concentrated on exhaling. Exhale and inhale three times respectively. Stress is laid on exhaling instead of inhaling.

4. Qi-Down-Pulling Method: After the deep exhaling and inhaling, move the hands away from the *Baihui* Point and lower them slowly from the top of the head to the *Shanzhong* Point with the middle fingers touching each other and the palms facing downward (see Figure 123). Now begin to pull down the *Qi* by taking long and deep exhalations, accompanied with waist-relaxing and leg-bending, with the backs of the hands facing each other and the fingers downward (see Figure 124). Stop the hands when the fingers reach the *Yinlingquan* Point (the inner side

below the knee) and stop exhaling, too (see Figure 125). The deep exhaling should be gentle, thin, even, long and calm.If the performer is not able to exhale so long, he can just exhale as long as possible. Then stand up and move the hands to *Dantian* with both palms turning toward the belly naturally.

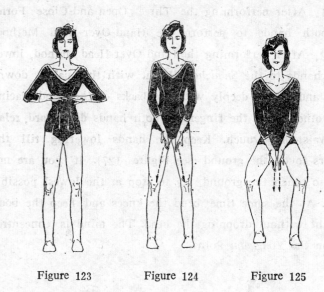

Figure 123   Figure 124   Figure 125

Repeat this three times in succession.

Ⅱ. **Conducting *Qi* to the *Zhongdu* Point**

1. Perform the Three Open-and-Close Form before lifting both hands to perform the Hand-Over-Head Method.

2. After performing the Hand-Over-Head Method, lower both hands to the *Shanzhong* Point with the palms down-wand and exhale deeply with the backs of both hands facing each other. Keep the fingers of both hands downward,

relax the waist and crouch. Keep lowering the hands till the fingers reach the *Zhongdu* Point (see Figure 126) and stop exhaling at the same time.

3. Stand up (the method is the same as mentioned before).

II. Conducting *Qi* to the *Yongquan* Point

1. After performing the Three Open-and-Close Form, lift both hands to perform the Hand-Over-Head Method.

2. After performing the Hand-Over-Head Method, lower both hands to the *Shanzhong* Point with the palms downward and exhale deeply with the backs of the hands facing each other. Keep the fingers of both hands downward, relax the waist and crouch. Keep the hands lowering till the fingers touch the ground (see Figure 127). If you are not able to touch the ground, try to stop at the lowest possible level. At the same time, bend the knees and keep the body upright without dropping the head. The mind is concentrated on the *Yongquan* Point.

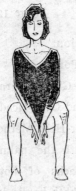
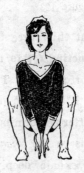

| Figure 126 | Figure 127 |

3. Stand up.

The above processes are called one round. Do three rounds altogether.

4. Do the Ending Form.

After conducting the *Qi* (vital energy) to the *Yongquan* Point, some performers may have a sense of breath-blocking. At this moment one can conduct the vital energy three *chi* deep into the ground and at once the breath-blocking sensation would disappear.

Only on the basis of practising the Breath-Regulating and *Qi*-Reenforcing Pattern and the Toe-Raised Transport and Conversion Pattern, can the Hypertension-Treating Pattern be effective in strengthening the original *yin* and regulate the vital energy and blood. So the vital energy will be converted. transported, smoothed and become abundant. Finally, the *yin* and *yang* are in the state of equilibrium and the blood pressure is regulated automatically. However, this *Qigong* method can only produce a short-term effect. To consolidate the results, the Blowing Method to Strengthen the Kidney must be added.

Chapter 3
The Massaging *Qigong* Pattern

The Massaging Pattern is a *Qigong* pattern that can be effective only on the basis of the five basic *Qigong* patterns of the Self-Controlled *Qigong* Therapy such as the Breath-Regulating and Qi-Reenforcing Pattern and the Toe-Raised Transport and Conversion Pattern. The Massaging Pattern requires that the performer emit his own *Qi*, and command the internal and external *Qi* to treat the diseased internal organs through massaging. Kidney Massage is the same as the Kidney-Massaging and Essence-Benefiting Pattern, which is not repeated here. The following are some massage methods for the internal organs.

Ⅰ. Heart Massage

1. Do the Starting Form.

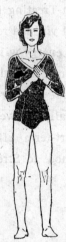

2. Put the left hand gently at the heart region below the left breast and put the right hand on top of the left hand (As for the female, put the right hand below the left breast) (see Figure 128). Massage twelve* circles leftward and massage another twelve circles in the opposite direction. Then do "point respiration" (three respirations for three massages). In the course of massaging, the hand can touch the skin gently or keep off the skin slightly according to the individual's manipulating strength (It is permissible to put the hand outside the clothes).

Figure 128

When massaging, the performer should focus his mind

---

* The number of circles is not a fixed figure. It can be increased or decreased by sixes.

on the heart so as to let the flow of the vital energy circle with the hand. Therefore, the blood circulates smoothly with the smooth flowing of the vital energy, thus promoting blood circulation and dispersing blood stasis and dredging the channels and collaterals.

3. Do the Ending Form.

The above processes are called one round. Do three rounds altogether.

Ⅱ. **Liver Massage**

1. Do the Starting Form.

2. Put the left hand (the right hand for the female) at the liver region below the right ribs and put the right hand (the left hand for the female) on top of the left (right) hand. Massage twelve circles leftward and massage another twelve circles rightward (see Figure 129). Then do "point respiration" (three respirations for three massages). In the course of massaging, the hand can touch the skin gently or keep off the skin slightly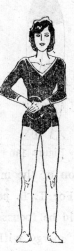

Figure 129

according to the individual's manipulating strength (It is permissible to put the hand outside the clothes).

When massaging, the performer should focus his mind on the liver, which serves to smooth and regulate the activities of vital energy, so as to make the vital energy flow inside the liver and conduct the liver-energy to flow downward.

3. Do the Ending Form.

Do three rounds. The number of circles for a round can be increased and decreased by sixes.

Ⅲ. **Lung Massage**

1. Do the Starting Form.

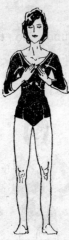

2. Put the two palms flatly on the lung region (see Figure 130) (Put them on the lesion region if it is known.) Massage twelve circles leftward and massage another twelve circles rightward. Then do "point respiration" (The method is the same as Heart Massage and Liver Massage).

When massaging, the mind is concentrated on the lung region. The lung cleanses the inspired air and keeps it flowing downward. The concentration of the mind helps this function of the lung's.

Figure 130

For T. B. patients with pulmonary holes. the mind should be focussed and concentrated so as to conduct the vital energy with mental control and to make the vital energy abundant. If the reaction is not favorable, the method of mentally downward pulling should be used, or the method tried from the beginning repeatedly if necessary.

3. Do the Ending Form.

4. Do this massage three times.

Ⅳ. **Spleen Massage and Stomach Massage**

For splenomegaly and dyspepsia, do the Spleen Massage.

For thoracic depression, abdominal distension, gastric ulcer, and gastritis, do the Stomach Massage.

1. Do the Starting Form.

2. Spleen Massage: Put the left hand (the right hand for the female) on the spleen region and put the right hand (left hand for the female) on top of the left hand. Massage twelve circles leftward and massage another twelve circles rightward (see Figure 131). Then, do "point respiration" with the mind concentrated on the spleen. The spleen is responsible for transport and conversion.So the flow of thoughts should follow the flowing Qi and the moving hand.

3. Stomach Massage

Put the left hand (right hand for the female) on the *Zhongwan* Point (the middle of the stomach) and put the right hand on top of the left hand (see Figure 132). Massage

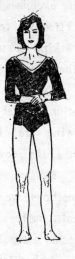
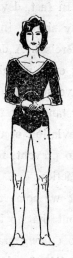

Figure 131   Figure 132

twelve circles leftward and rightward respectively. Then, do "point respiration". The stomach is responsible for receiving and holding food and functions to digest food. So the mind should be concentrated in such a way as to make the stomach feel a sense of warmth.

4. Do the Ending Form.

Do this massage three times.

Chapter 4
Methods to Prevent, Rectify and Control Deviations in *Qigong* Practice

Many people worry about the deviations in *Qigong* exercises. In fact, deviations in *Qigong* exercises are inevitable. They show, in a way, the effective reactions of *Qigong* exercises. A deviation means a kind of uncomfortableness or even morbid reaction. So the *Qigong* practitioners should have some knowledge of the principles of *Qigong* and understand how to prevent deviations. What will you do if a deviation occurs? The following are the specific methods to prevent, rectify and control the deviations in *Qigong* practice.

Before we come to the specific methods, we would like to point out that to keep in good health is the foundation of life. So *Qigong* practice should become a regular part of a person's life. In the prologue to his book "How to Keep

Fit", Zhang Zhan points out "the principle of keeping fit mainly consists of the following nine points: ① not wasting the essence of life; ② cherishing the vital energy; ③ building a good shape and a healthy constitution; ④ doing the breathing and physical exercise (daoyin); ⑤ speech; ⑥ food; ⑦ sexual life ⑧ medical care; ⑨ avoiding the taboos." Of the above-mentioned nine points, only four are related to Qigong. The rest all belong to life activities. This shows clearly the great importance of having a regular life habit, which the Qigong practitioners should not overlook.

I. Deviation-Preventing Method

1. The mind should be free from over-concentration or aberrations. If a beginner simply acquires a hot feeling in a certain part of his body after a short period of Qigong practice and he would try to guide his thought to go through the "three passes", the Ren Channel and the Du Channel and seek hallucination (This is called "painstaking effort" in Qigong), then he would have "disorder of consciousness" or even "mental confusion", that is, deviation caused by "painstaking effort". The performer should understand that Qigong has its own laws. Smooth channels and collaterals are developed naturally in the course of Qigong practice. It can not be accomplished in one morning. So we do not encourage the performer "to conduct Qi with mental power", which can lead to disorders such as head-shaking and shoulder-shrugging, waist-twisting and back-hunching, hand and leg quivering, stumbling and staggering, uncon-

trolled crying or even opisthotonos and stiff and twisted extremities. The performer sometimes even goes as far as to lose self-control. So when doing *Qigong* exercises, mental power should not be used at random and quiescence should be considered as the dominant factor. Quiescence helps to tranquilize the mind and a tranquilized mind helps recuperate and strengthen the health.

2. Control the function of the six senses and do not get disturbed by the environment. To control the six senses means to control the eyes, the nose, the tongue, the ears, the body and the mind. It is a hard job for a person not to hear the sounds in the environment, but he should be able to control himsef so as not to worry over the sounds and noises in the environment. On the contrary, he should be able to turn the noises into something that he is delighted to hear. After a long period of practice, the performer not only can resist the disturbance of noises and obtain tranquility among noises, but also avoid being fascinated by the five notes of traditional Chinese music, the five colors or the five flavors. Not being fascinated by the five colors means to keep the eyes half-closed and look horizontally into the far distance but see nothing. When practising the quiescent *Qigong* exercises, the performer can have an inner object, which means not a single object to be seen in the surroundings. The inner object can be "observed" only when the performer looks within himself. It should not be sought with effort. He should not be attracted by the beauty or have any evil thought. Not to be fascinated by the five

flavors means that during *Qigong* exercises, if there is any fragrant smell of flower, scent, wine or meat, the performer should not be fascinated or carried away by them. He should remain indifferent to them.

3. Prevent fatigue. When doing *Qigong* exercises, the performer should avoid fatigue and should take a break for rest as soon as he feels tired. In his daily life activities, a *Qigong* practitioner should also prevent overtiredness, guard against internal injury and maintain an appropriate balance between work and rest, And the most important of all is to avoid excessive sexual intercourse. The purpose of "invigorating the body fluid to promote essential substance" and invigorating the essential substance to promote vital energy" in practising *Qigong* is to make both the essential substance and vital energy abundant. The essential substance is the basis of the spirits. The spirits perish at the exhaustion of vital energy. So a person must not seek the temporary pleasure of sexual life at the expense of his lifelong happiness. Those who suffer from diseases should be more careful about it. They should suspend sexual acts for the first three months of their *Qigong* practice and be temperate afterwards.

4. Guard against exogenous evils. The heat-evil reduces marrow and the cold-evil damages the spleen and the muscles. The practitioner should change clothes as the weather changes. He should neither pracise *Qigong* in the draught nor practise it in the wind, or rain or under the scorching sun, or when there is thunder and lightning. When

the performer is moist with sweat after *Qigong* exercises, he should not sit in the wind, or it will be harmful to his health.

5. Be careful with the functional activities of vital energy. To practise *Qigong*, the performer must pay enough attention to the functional activities of vital energy.

(1) Before practising, remove the obstacles that may affect the functional activities of vital energy. For example, wear loose clothes and do not wear a tight waist belt, watch band, shoelaces, garters, or unduly tight or high-heeled shoes. Relieve yourself before practising.Do not practise when you are very hungry or very full, greatly surprised, greatly angry or overjoyed.

(2) You should keep calm when practising and turn a deaf ear to whatever surprises or disturbances that occur in the surroundings or inside the body. You must have a fully prepared mind against any sudden sounds in the environment. For example, when your mind is tranquilized, you hear people greeting you, people shouting or crying, or sounds of vehicles and sounds of collision between stones or bricks. Even if you are shocked, you should control yourself and restore your mind to the normal state of calmness. If your mind is disturbed because of surprise, you can perform the Open-and-Close at the Two *Dantians* immediately. Usually you can get calmed down after you perform it four times. If not, you should keep on performing it` until you are calmed down. Otherwise, sequelae may result from it (In addition to the Open-and-Close at the Two *Dantians*,

the Method of Promoting Vital Energy by *Daoyin* may also be used). For the purpose of safety, a quiet place should be selected for *Qigong* exercises. If you are called by someone during *Qigong* exercises, you should remain calm and at ease and you do not have to respond. Be sure not to get angry because of being startled. Otherwise, disorders of vital energy and pulse may occur.

It is a common phenomenon that during *Qigong* exercises, there occur the Eight Sensations: "bigness, smallness, lightness, heaviness, coldness, hotness, itching and numbness". These sensations show the different states of the vital energy—either in motion or being blocked. Whichever case it may be, the performer should persist in practising with confidence. Any hesitation will lead to confusion, which can affect the *Qigong* technique as well as the result.

When practising *Qigong* in the sitting position, the performer should have his feet touching firmly on the ground instead of suspending them in midair, no matter he is sitting on a chair or on the edge of a bed. Otherwise, he will have swollen feet and lumbago (due to the stagnation of blood) or hallucination which can cause him to fall down to the ground and spoil the entire exercise.

When hallucination occurs during *Qigong* exercises, the performer should not induce himself into the illusion and allow himself to be carried away by the emotions. If hallucination occurs, the performer should go on practising peacefully and with pleasure. Then press his hands at *Dantian*

223

to end the exercises. He should not be sentimental at the illusion—being sad or joyful, or speeding up his breath, which will interrupt the breathing rhythm and lead to deviations.

To practise Qigong, the performer should select a proper Qigong pattern that fits his illness— to tonify or to purge, and work out a rational programme that suits his case. He should never practise at random. Otherwise, pathological changes may occur. The principles for tonification and purgation are: The right is for tonification and the left is for purgation. So the diseases that require purgation are treated by performing from left to right; the diseases that require tonification are treated by performing from right to left. The inward-turning hands are for tonification and the outword-turning hands are for purgation; the upward-moving hands, which can regulate the yang-energy to rise, are inclined to toninfy, and the downward-moving hands, which can pull the yang-energy down, are inclined to purge; open eyes are for purgation and closed eyes are for tonification. The performer should apply these princlples according to the symptoms of his disease. The pithy formula and the silent recitation also have the functions of tonification and purgation. Roughly speaking, the second tone is for tonification and the first tone is for purgation.

6. If any saliva comes out during Qigong exercises, swallow it down in three portions, swallowing it down mentally to Dantian. It will be beneficial to your health

if you perspire a little, but you should avoid the wind. Stop practising if you perspire profusely, for it is liable to hurt the *yin*. So do not practise *Qigong* in wet clothes. Do not go to the toilet within half an hour after the practising in order to avoid the conditional reflex that you feel like going to the toilet the moment you begin to do *Qigong* exercises. This can also help avoid the leakage of vital energy.

II. Deviation-Rectifying Method

Deviation will occur if the performer is not careful. If a deviation occurs, it must be rectified. To rectify a deviation, the performer must make clear the cause and suit the remedy to the case no matter whether he rectifies the deviation himself or he has the deviation rectified with the help of others. Generally speaking, a deviation is usually caused by the following five factors: life activities, postural changes, breathing methods, mental activities and disturbance of *Qigong* exercises. So a deviation is to be rectified in these five aspects.

1. Check up Your Life Activities: Try to make clear everything that is connected with your work, housework, life activities, balance between work and rest and so on other than *Qigong* practice itself. On this basis find out the correct rectifying method.

2. Postural *Daoyin*: To check up a deviation in postural *daoyin*) is to see "whether relaxation is achieved"; "whether the postures are correct"; "whether tonification or purgation is appropriate". As far as the Self-Controlled *Qigong* Therapy is concerned, the eighteen basic steps of mo-

vements mentioned before are the most fundamental requirements. The Breath-Regulating and Qi-Reenforcing Pattern and the Toe-Raised Transport and Conversion Pattern are both performed on this basis. Even the *Qigong* patterns in sitting position are based on the relaxation of these requirements. Other *Qigong* patterns have their own specific requirements, but they all have a basic law. So when a deviation occurs, the performer should check it up by himself or with the help of others according to the basic law. A beginner is subject to some disorders because of his incorrect postures. For example, he may have disorders such as headache, dizziness, neckache, stiff nape, pain in the shoulder and the back because he fails to relax himself or stretches his back or hollows his chest too hard. Stiff or painful neck is usually caused by forceful efforts in suspending the head. Eye distension results from fixed looking during the exercises. Lumbago or pain in the hips results from the failure in waist-relaxation due to the failure in hip-relaxation, or results from the twisting of the waist without relaxing the hips or from the forceful twisting of the waist. Abdominal flatulence or distension results from the forceful pulling-in of the stomach or too much concentration of the mind. Swollen and painful anus and even dry stool result from forceful raising of the anus. Sore knee results from crouching too low or over-bending of the knees. The cause of the pain in the heels is due to the excessive body weight shifted on the heels during walking. Heelache may also occur if the performer focuses his mind on the heels instead of on the toe tips or if he knocks the heels against the ground. Sexual excess or kidney-asthenia is another cause for the pain in the heels.

So the performer should distinguish *yin* and *yang* as well as asthenia and sthenia in the up-and-down movement of the hands during *Qigong* exercises. The palms of the hands should face the body; the opposite direction can easily cause diarrhoea and deficiency of vital energy. If the hands move outward from the kidney regions on the sides in the manner of making circles, lumbago will be caused. The Method to Strengthen the Kidney requires the performer to step out with the right foot first, otherwise, lumbago may occur. If the fingers of the hands move up to point at the chest, it will cause tightness in the chest. If they point obliquely at the neck and face, it will cause dizziness, nausea and edema of the face to those who are sensitive to their channels and collaterals. If the performer feels that his lower limbs are too heavy to lift during the exercises, he can correct it by thinking of the *Ba hui* Poin. If he feels that his body is too light and unsteady, he can think of the *Yongquan* Point in each of the soles.

The performer should avoid violent activities such as running immediately after *Qigong* exercises so as to prevent the wrong flowing of the vital energy or pain in the legs.

If there occur deviations in the postures, review the eighteen methods in standing position first, and then review the other *Qigong* patterns. To rectify deviations, the performer can practise the Method to Strengthen the Lung so as to invigorate the flowing of the internal vital energy and rectify its disorder. If this method does not work, the Relaxed and Quiescent Qi-Regulating Pattern (with a stick) can be performed.

3. Breathing *Daoyin*: Deviations in breathing often result from the wrong performance of the Three Deep Exhaling and Inhaling Method of the Starting Form. The performer shou dcheck whether the exhalation is long enough when crouching and whether there is enough leeway left when exhaling on the basis of checking relaxation and quiescence. Excessive crouching can easily cause pain in the legs. Toolong exhalings or trying to expel all the air out can easily cause shortness of breath. To inhale the moment the tongue touches the upper gum, the performer not only can not breathe in any air but also can suffer from shortness of breath, tightness in the chest and abdominal distension. Both exhaling and inhaling should be gentle, thin, even and long. When standing up after inhaling, he should breathe properly and naturally to regulate the breath and should not hold the breath (note: The performer can hold his breath only when he is skilled in *Qigong* practice). It is best to inhale at a little below the *Shangen* Point. The Blowing Method of the Breath-Regulating and Qi-Reenforcing Pattern requires breathing through the middle bridge of the nose. Inappropriate breathing may cause headache, tightness in the chest and even discomfort in the heart. To perform the Two-Inhaling and One-Exhaling Method of the Breath-Regulating and Qi-Reenforcing Pattern, the perfor-

mer must not connect the two inhalings into one. Otherwise tightness in the chest will occur. The exhaling should be fast instead of dragging on, or it will cause general weakness and fatigue. It is best to turn the inhaling and exhaling into natural abdominal paradoxical inhaling and paradoxical exhaling, that is, when inhaling through the nose, pull in the navel as if to lift the body with two contractions following two inhalings, and when exhaling, blow out through the nose as if to expel half of the inhaled air and keep the rest inside as if a rushing force entering Middle *Dantian*. If this method is properly applied, the symptoms such as tightness in the chest, shortness of breath and abdominal distenstion will disappear. Because breath belongs to the Lung Channel, the Blowing Method to Strengthen the Lung can also be applied to rectify deviations. So long as breath is well regulated, there will be no problem about sinking the vital energy to *Dantian*.

4. Mental *Daoyin*: Deviations caused by mental *daoyin* can be rectified by postural *daoyin*, however, they should be rectified mainly by mental control in the following aspects:

(1) Deviations in mental *daoyin* are caused mainly by overthinking. They canebe rectified by counting numbers—using one thought to replace the many thoughts. True, it is impossible for a beginner to get absolutely tranquilized. It is even difficult for a veteran performer to tranquilize his mind to the extent of "having no thought". Actually "having no thought" can cause "painstaking effort for empti-

ness", which is also forbidden. Some people think that counting numbers is too simple a method and they are not interested in it.So they try to concentrate their minds on an object in the surroundings. This is, in fact, subject to deviations. It is only after a certain period of practice can a performer begin to concentrate his mind on an object in the surroundings, but he has to abide by the following rules strictly:

Concentrate the mind on a motionless instead of moving object: For example, a hypertension patient can concentrate his mind on still lake water, but not on the surging sea.

Concentrate the mind on a near object instead of a far one: For example, a patient of liver trouble can concentrate his mind on a pine tree nearby so as to have it at his beck and call. If the performer is at the Temple of Heaven in Beijing, and his mind is absorbed in concentration of a pine tree of the Huangshan Mountain in Anhui Province, which is far away, he has to trace in imagination to the object with painstaking efforts. So when anything unexpected crops up, it will be very difficult for him to end the exercises. As a result, his mind will be wandering and his spirits will be low.

Concentrate the mind on a familiar instead of an unfamiliar object: Like the rule to concentrate on a near instead of a far object, concentrate on something you are familiar with and not on anything that is strange to you, on something you like and not on anything you have no affec-

tion for. Otherwise, it will cause estrangement in your af-
ections and uneasiness in your mind.

Suit the methods to the cases: Patients with hypertension (including other high indexes such as high transaminase) should concentrate their minds on a low place instead
of a high one. Patients with hypotension (including other
low indexes such as low haemochrome) should concentrate
their minds on a high instead of a low place. T. B. patients should concentrate on white and light things (e.g.
white clouds, floss silk). Patients with spleen and stomach
diseases should concentrate on yellow and unfurled things
(e. g., yellow chrysanthemum, dahlia). Patients with hepatic diseases should concentrate on green plants (e. g., pine,
cypress). Patients with heart trouble should concentrate on
things of red color, but red color is too energetic and its
tone is unstable. So it makes it diffcult for the performer
to get tranquilized. Therefore, the purple or pink lotus is
preferrable. Patients with kidney diseases should concentrate
on things of black color. But black color, is depressing, and
can easily cause the kidney-energy to sink, which can put
the performer into low spirits. This is unfavorable to the
disease. So for patients with kidney diseases, it is prefera-
ble to choose things of purple color and strong articles such
as handicrafts of sandalwood.

When deciding On an external object, it is forbidden
for the performer to choose human beings, his own work
or evil and obscene affairs. The performer is also forbidden
to think of from one thing to another, back and forth

without stopping.

The deviations caused by mental activities can be rectified by choosing appropriate external objects according to the above-mentioned taboos. If a person is mentally depressed, he should not do any *Qigong* exercise before he gets rid of his depression. Otherwise, it will cause headache, tightness in the chest, or even shock for severe cases. The solution to this problem is to lead the vital energy downward along the channels. If the performer fails to do it himself, he can ask other people for help or use the Hypertension-Treating Pattern.

(2) Another deviation in mental *daoyin* is caused by the words and sentences that the performer utters. Some people like to utter the Chinese character "*fó*". This character is in the rising tone, which can easily cause the vital energy to rise. If the vital energy rises the moment the performer gets tranquilized, it will cause dizziness and nausea. So in this case, the performer should stop exercising. If the performer changes to utter the character "*fǔ*" in the third (falling-rising) tone, the vital energy will descend and the performer can get tranquilized easily. Some other people utter the sentence: "Xiongkou shuchang qixie tong (If the pit of the stomach feels comfortable, the vital energy and blood will flow freely)". This sentence is a good message, which should cause no problems. But as it too many rising and falling-rising tones it contains too much motivity. And moreover, it expresses too strong a desire for recovering, so after it is uttered silently, there will occur symptoms such

as dizziness and slight fever, tightness in the chest and leg weakness, foul breath and bloody stool. These symptoms can not be relieved by medicine. However, some people have succeeded in rectifying such deviations by doing the Open-and-Close at the Two *Dantians* to regulate the excess of *yang*. This shows that if the performer selects anything at random for mental concentration without understanding the theory of *Qigong*, he can easily get into trouble.

(3) Deviations in an individual's mental activities should be rectified by controlling the mental activities and a performer should well understand the principle that spirits are the commander of vital energy. Spirits are mental activities, which decide all the individual's activities. Deviations in mental activities should be regulated and controlled by the individual's own strength. The main method is to calm oneself down and do the Breath-Regulating and Qi-Reenforcing Pattern, the Open-and-Close at the Two *Dantians* and the Open-and-Close at the Three *Dantians*.

5. *Daoyin* for the Disturbed *Qigong* Exercise: Most often when a performer gets startled, he is already in the state of tranquility. He is either disturbed by an unexpected sound or by unexpected happenings. To avoid such disturbances, the performer should be careful when choosing an environment and a site for *Qigong* exercises. When exercising, a safe and preventive warning should be given to the brain. By doing so, even when the performer is startled, there will be no problems caused. If he is not prepared mentally, when he is startled, the deviations will be very dif-

ficult to rectify. The following are some methods to prevent the performer from being startled:

(1) It is absolutely forbidden for the performer to open his eyes when he is startled while doing *Qigong* exercises. If he opens his eyes, the disturbed vital energy will be thrown into confusion and the stagnated vital energy will cause deviations which are hard to rectify. After a performer is startled, if he goes on exercising with his eyes shut as if nothing had happened, he can restore his mind to the normal state by guiding the vital energy along the routes of channels to bring it back to the channels.

(2) The specific method of guiding the vital energy along the routes of channels is to keep the eyes shut when startled and immediately do the Open-and-Close at the Two *Dantians* (possibly a number of times). The two *Dantians* refer to the *Yintang* Point and the *Qihai* Point. Raise the hands to the lower jaw and breathe in with a hissing sound as if inhaling a mouthful of cold air. Following the inhaled air, the hands move up to the *Yintang* Point and do the Opening while breathing out slowly. Repeat this Open-and-Close at the Two *Dantians* four times. If the performer still feels uncomfortable, he can work up to eight times to solve the problem.

6. The Method to Rectify Deviations with a Stick: The *Qigong* method with a stick of the Relaxed and Quiescent Qi-Regulating Pattern is a perfect deviation-rectifying method that can dredge the channels and collaterals and promote the flow of vital energy and blood. This method is very effec-

234

tive in rectifying deviations caused by inappropriate tonification or purgation. When doing this deviation-rectifying exercise, rotate the stick outward for purgation and inward is for tonification. More practice of this method not only can rectify the deviations but also can help promote the vital energy.

7. The Blowing Method to Strengthen the Lung: This is also a useful method to rectify deviations. When a performer feels uncomfortable after *Qigong* exercises, he can practise this method for 20 minutes. The performer should have his whole body relaxed, exercising leisurely, with carefree ness and with a smile on his face.

8. The Carefree Method: For those people whose deviations are prolonged and hard to rectify or have been half-rectified, this method can be practised. This method is a carefree method. The performer walks casually as if half drunk, touching the ground with the toetips and the *Yongquan* Points, and with the whole body relaxed. Practise this method 1-2 times a day.

Those who suffer from tightness in the chest or abdominal distension can enunciate the sound "ha" six to nine times for a course according to the word-pronouncing method. The above-mentioned deviation-rectifying method is to be chosen in consideration of the kinds and stages of the specific disease. It must not be used at random.

Ⅱ. Deviation-Controlling Method

When the performer has made his *Qigong* exercises function automatically and can not be stopped, a part of his

235

body often keeps moving for two or three hours, or even a whole day, which is very exhausting. In this case, it should be controlld in the following ways:

1. Induce the Mover by Words: Advise the performer by saying: "Violent movement is not as good as gentle movement; gentle movement is not as good as no movement; it is time you ended your exercises for a rest". Repeated advising like this can help him prepare mentally for a stop. This method is usually effective.

2. Stop the Mover by Command: Direct the mover to put his left hand at Middle *Dantian*. If he is obedient, he will also put his right hand on top of his left hand himself. If not, the helper can take the mover's left hand, with his own left hand, to press *Dantian* and strike the mover's gate of life three times with his right fist (or palm). This can help the mover to end the exercise. (This is rather a compulsive method.)

3. If the above-mentioned method does not help, the helper can direct the mover to turn the right foot inward with the tiptoe pointing at the heel of the left foot. If the mover fails to do it himself, the helper should take the mover's left hand with his own right hand and with his foot push the tiptoe of the mover's right foot to point at the heel of the left heel. That will help the mover to end the exercise. The helper can also touch the mover's *Tai-chong* Point (between the big and the second toes) with dagger fingers.

Book IV

QIGONG PRESCRIPTIONS
FOR SYMPTOMS

Chapter 1
Introduction

Before giving treatment to a patient, a doctor of Chinese traditional medicine first of all forms a judgement of the locus and nature of the ailment by analysing, synthesizing and summing up all the data gathered through the 4 methods of examination (observation, listening and smelling inquiring, pulse feeling and palpitation) in accordance with the patient's pathological condition. This is called "determination of treatment based on the differentiation of symptomps and signs". But in the case of *Qigong* therapy, the patient can be taught to do the breathing exercises for all the diagnosed or undiagnosed chronic or difficult cases so long as the asthenia and sthenia syndromes are differentiated. Nevertheless, in differentiating the eight principal syndromes (*yin* and *yang*, superficies and interior, cold and heat, asthenia and sthenia) an experienced *Qigong* instructor is sure to have detailed analysis and study of the symptoms of the patient.

Superficies and interior refer to the locations of ailments. The superficies-syndrome indicates that the illness is on the surface or outer part of the body while the interior-syndrome indicates that the illness is in the internal part of the body. Generally speaking, chronic diseases belong to the

239

interior-syndrome in most cases. Cold and heat refer to the nature of an ailment. "An excess of *yang* brings about heat-syndrome while an excess of *yin* brings about cold-syndrome". The cold-syndrome often has such symptoms as adversion to cold and desire for warmth, deadly cold hands and feet, pale complexion and loose stool or the attenuation of physical mechanism. The heat-syndrome often has the following symptoms: fever and desire for coolness, flushed face and ears, dry mouth and tongue, and dry stool. Asthenia and sthenia are the basis on which the state of healthy energy and the degree of seriousness of an illness are differentiated. The asthenia-syndrome is often seen with patients who have listlessness, feebleness, emaciation, shortness of breath, spontaneous perspiration and night sweat, frequency or incontinence of feces and urine, poor appetite, palpitation and insomnia, and numbness of hands and feet. The sthenia-syndrome is often seen with patients who have a feeling of fullness in the chest, abdomen, hypochondrium and gastric cavity, constipation and obstruction of mictuaration. *Yin* and *yang* are the general principles. Cold, interior and asthenia belong to the *yin*-syndrome while heat, superficies and sthenia belong to the *yang*-syndrome.

According to self-controlled *Qigong* therapy, diseases can mainly be put into two categories: the sthenia-syndrome and the asthenia-syndrome.

The sthenia-syndrome includes such diseases as cancer, tumour, lump and liver cirrhosis, which are characteristic of stagnation of vital energy and blood stasis, accumulation and stagnation of heat and cold.

The asthenia-syndrome includes diseases of the debilitated superficies and interior involving the patient's vital organs such as the heart, liver, spleen, lung, kidney and the pericardium, gall-bladder, stomach, large intestine, small intestine, bladder and the triple warmer. Chronic diseases which are marked by blockage of the channel passage, disorder of vital energy and blood, breakdown of even balance of *yin* and *yang*, are also included in asthenia-syndrome.

Chapter 2
Prescriptions for and Case Studies of Some Common Diseases

I. Prescriptions for and Case Studies of Cardiovascular Diseases

As the heart controls the arteries and veins, coronary heart disease is a disease in which the patient's coronary arteries are hardened. Congenital heart disease, rheumatic heart disease, organic pathological changes of heart, nervous malfunctioning of the heart, arteriosclerosis of the brain, myocarditis, vasculitis and hypertension can all be put into the category of cardiovascular diseases.

The major *Qigong* patterns used to treat cardiovascular diseases include: The Blowing Method to Strengthen the

Kidney, the Blowing Method to Strengthen the Heart, the Toe-Raised Transport and Conversion Pattern and the Head-Massaging and Mind-Tranquilizing Pattern.

Moreover, for patients with rheumatism and patients with vasculitis, the Relaxed and Quiescent *Qi*-Regulating Pattern should be added. For patients with insomnia, the Kidney-Massaging and Essence-Benefiting Pattern should be added.

Pronounce the sounds of the Chinese charac ters "zheng" (tone 1) and Zhěng (tone 3) as a pair for seven times. To start, pronounce them 3 times and continue to pronounce them up to the seventh time if no untoward effect occurs.

Patients with cardiovascular diseases should also do the hear tmassage once in the morning and once in the evening.

Case No. 1

Patient: Yang, male, 47, works at the Beijing Special Steel Works.

Patient had constant palpitation, general weakness, pale lips and grey face. He was examined in the factory hospital in March and diagnosed as having sinus arrhythmia, repeated ventricular premature systole. After ten weeks of *Qigong* exercise, patient gained physical strength and suddenly became optimistic in mood. Palpitation also dropped So patient became more confident of the effect of *Qigong* therapy and went on practising it every day. Two months later, his electrocardiogram became normal.

Case No. 2

Patient: Fan, female, 43, works as a physician in the Taixi Hospital, Qingdo.

For 25 years patient has suffered from rheumatic heart disease with valve pathological changes in the bicuspid aortic valve, complicated by paroxysmal tachycardia of the upper ventricle. During the past 10 years and more, intermittent pre-excitation syndrome and functional prostration in the sino-atrial bundle frequently occurred beyond control. The physical method of pressing the eyeballs was applied to ease off the symptoms. But repeated recurrences followed day after day, year after year. Her health was seriously threatened.

On the night of Jan. 20, 1981, after repeated recurrences, she had the cornea of her left eye broken accidentally and the sight of the eye was lost. Now physiotherapy could no longer be used to ease off the disease, she had to be hospitalized. Still, arrested heart beat occured several times after that. Later she began to practise *Qigong* with the help of her doctors. On the first day, she could hardly stand on her feet, her heart beating fast, her eyes swimming and her legs shivering. She went on practising by supporting herself on the rails. Only after many breaks and rests could she manage to practise for one or two minutes. She even felt worse after the exercise and her doctor had to give her intravenous drip for hormones. However, the patient did not lose hope. She persevered in practising the breathing technique. Gradually, she could stand on her feet by herself for 2 minutes, 5 mintes, 10 minutes and even an hour. A month later, she felt much better both mentally and physically. In addition to a better appetite and sleep, she gained some physical strength and became more energetic; her palpitation decreased and arrhythmia corrected. Four months later, she gave up all the Western drugs, only taking some Chinese traditional medical herbs occasionally. The function of her sino-atrial bundle was basically restored. Her heart beat was 60~70/min, regular and forceful. At present the patient can do *Qigong* exercise continuously for two hours without feeling tired.

Case No. 3

Patient: Xu, female, 48, works in the Capital Hospital.

Patient's condition is complicated. Eight years ago, in 1973 she stopped working for a complete rest. In 1960, she contracted dropsy and in 1963 she was sick with rheumatic arthritis with a slight fever of around 37.8 degrees centigrade and erythrocyte sedimentation rate (ESR) 48mm/h. In 1964 she suffered from hepatitis with such symptoms as pain in the hepatic region, nausea and abdominal distension, poor appetite. The diagnosis was confirmed as chronic hepatitis by liver puncture. In 1968 she had ectopia of the endometrium and in 1973 she suffered from "morbid sinus syndrome" with the following clinic manifestations: bradycardia, arrhythmia, heartbeat 30~40/min complicated by "sinus suspension of the heartbeat" and "sinus reclusive heartbeat", dizziness all day long, tightness in the chest, shortness of breath and palpitation, angina pectoris, insomnia, and poor appetite. Patient could hardly take care of herself and was thus hospitalized more than 20 times. She was believed to suffer from deficiency of the heart function and a cardiac pacemaker had to be used to keep her heart beating. So the patient lost all hope.

After two months of *Qigong* practice, the invalid took a favourable turn in her sleep, appetite, mental state and physical strength. She could now manage to take care of herself in daily affairs. Moreover, her feces began to take shape; her edema subsided; her blood pressure became normal; her body weight dropped by 10 *jin* and the heart arrests and retrograde heartbeats disappeared·

Case No. 4

Patient: Wang, female 44, is a doctor at a convalescent home in Qingdao.

Patient had been ill with hypertension for more than 10 years prior to her *Qigong* practice. During the last three years, her blood pressure often went up as high as 200/130 mm.Hg, with minimum pressure at around 160/110mm.Hg. She had been on depressors, but her blood pressure never dropped to the normal level. Her hypertension was usually complicated by symptoms such as palpitation, tightness and oppression in the chest, feeling of fullness in the head and hypomnesia. Normal as her electrocardiogram was, there was diastolic murmur in her precardium. And her electrocardiogram suggests ventricular hypertrophy while the thoracoscopy suggests expansion of her heart. Besides, she had chronic hepatitis and some other diseases.

Patient has insisted on doing *Qigong* exercise for 1—1.5 hours every day ever since she started. About one month later, her condition improved obviously. Some subjective symptoms such as palpitation, fatigue and feeling of tightness and oppression in the chest disappeared completely. What was prominent was that she felt happy and was full of vigour. Her blood pressure and the hepatic function became normal.

Ⅱ. **Prescriptions for and Case Studies of Liver Diseases**

The liver stores blood and generates wind. Many liver diseases may have the following symptoms: blood failing to imbue the liver, excessive liver-fire flaring up, a bad taste in the mouth and coughing up blood, dry and astringent feeling inboth eyes, eyes russet in colour, distension in the chest and hypochondrium, numbness and quivering in the limbs and general weakness.

The major *Qigong* patterns used to treat liver diseases include: The Blowing Method to Strengthen the Kidney, The Blowing Method to Strengthen the Liver, the Spleen and the Lung as well as the Relaxed and Quiescent Qi-Regulating Pattern.

For patients with liver diseases complicated by hypertension, the Toe-Raised Transport and Conversion Pattern should be added.

For patients whose liver diseases have affected the spleen and who feel uncomfortable in the stomach, the Toe-Raised Transport and Conversion Pattern should be added.

For patients with liver diseases complicated by ocular diseases, the Head-Massaging and Mind-Tranquilizing Pattern should be added.

For patients with liver diseases complicated by arthritis and spasm of hands and feet, the Relaxed and Quiescent Qi-Regulating Pattern should be practised at least twice a day.

Patients with liver diseases pronounce the sound of the Chinese character "guo" four times first and then, continue to pronounce the same sound up to the eighth time when adapted to it. And in addition, the massage of the hepatic region should also be practised.

Case No. 1

Patient: Huang, male, 53, is an army man.

In 1963, the patient was hospitalized for hepatitis. He was discharged upon recovery, but may recurrences followed. The indexes for each recurrence are roughly as follows:

1. Transaminase: about 500 units.

2. TTT (thymol turbidity test): over 20 units.

3. Flocculation test: +++

4. HAA(hepatitis-associated antigen): +

5 Paste-like feces

6. Dull pain in the hepatic region, restlessness and general weakness.

With a painful experience of the disease, the patient persisted in practising *Qigong* every day. He practised the Breath-Regulating and Qi-reenforcing Pattern, the Toe-Raised Transport and Conversion Pattern, Massage of the Hepatic Region and the Deep Exhaling in Sitting Position every morning (before 7 o'clock). In the evening, he practised the Toe-Raised Transport and Conversion Pattern as well as the

247

Massage of the Hepatic Regoin. Two months later the patient's condition improved obviously. All the indexes of the disease were changing for the better. The following is a comparison between the patient's condition before he took up *Qigong* practice and that after two months' practice:

item	before practice	after practice
transaminase	normal	normal
TTT	17	5
flocculation test	+	−
general symptoms	lack of strength, inclination for sleep	energetic; lightness in walking; no inclination for sleep or bed rest

Case No. 2

Patient: Xu, female, 35, works in a factory of semiconductor appliances.

With a case history of three years of rheumatoid arthritis, the patient received treatment in several large hospitals, but still had had no distinctive improvement in her condition. Besides, her spleen and stomach were damaged as a consequence of the side effects of the drugs. She had a severe pain in her joints which were swollen and partly deformed. Consequently, she could not take care of herself in her daily life activities. When her condition got serious, she could not get up from bed, her neck was stiff and her jaw could not move freely. Later she received treatment in the Chongwen District Hospital of Traditional Chinese Med-

248

icine. After she took the traditional Chinese medicine "Bashfeng" for some time, her condition improved preliminarily. Then she began to learn *Qigong* exercise. Six days later she began to have the "sensation of *Qi*". After a fortnight, the pain in her knees subsided and three months later she felt no pain in either knee. She was able to walk like a healthy person in fine weather. She could even climb up to the 4th floor without the help of a stick.

Ⅲ. **Prescriptions for and Case Studies of Pneumonopathy**

As the lung controls the vital energy, diseases of the lung usually have symptoms such as shortness of breath, panting and coughing. Tracheitis, bronchitis, asthma and pulmonary tuberculosis are examples of such diseases.

The major *Qigong* pattern used to treat pneumonopathy is the Breath-Regulating and Qi-Reenforcing Pattern. Patients without palpitation may not use the Blowing Method to Strengthen the Heart.

For patients who have a feeling of oppression in the chest and patients whose hearts are affected, the Open-and-Close Method at the Three *Dantians* should be added.

For Patients with abundant expectoration and poor appetite, the Toe-Raised Transport and Conversion Pattern should be added.

For patients with insomnia, the Toe-Raised Transport and Conversion Pattern and the Head-massaging and Mind-Tranquilizing Pattern should also be added.

For patients with breathing noises, the Relaxed and

Quiescent Qi-Regulating Pattern should be added.

Patients with pulmonary diseases should pronounce the Chinese character "shang" for expulsion of air. Pronounce nine times altogether: first three times, if the patient d es not feel uncomfortable, he can work up to six times, and gradually to nine times. Massage of the Pulmonary Region should also be added.

Case No. 1

Patient: female, 62.

With a case history of 30 years of asthma, the patient visited many hospitals and received every possible treatment, but no improvement was effected. Her condition was very bad and she often caught cold. When she walked, she always panted or gasped for breath, her heart palpitating, her head swimming, and her eyes dim-sighted. She could not fall asleep at night without the help of hypnotics and asthma pills.Also she had gastric trouble with symptoms such as acid regurgitation, stagnation of intestinal gas, belching, poor appetite. listlessness and pale complexion.

After one month's *Qigong* exercice, her condition improved, both mentally and physically, and she had a better appetite, too. She could fall asleep without taking hypnotics or asthma pills. After three months' practice, her asthma no longer recurred, her gastric trouble disappeared and she rarely caught cold. Now she is full of vigour and vitality. She has rosy cheeks and has also gained weight.

Case No. 2

Patient: Zhang, female, 25, a worker in a broadcast

equipment factory.

In Jan. 1977, the patient expectorated blood. At a hospital of pulmonary tuberculosis, she was diagnosed as having "infiltrative pulmonary tuberculosis at the stage of dissolution in the upper right lung". After 6 months' hospitalization for treatment, her doctor believed that she must be operated on. The operation was not performed, because she was too nervous. So she was discharged from the hospital with the pulmonary cavity in her lung.

When she learned that *Qigong* could cure diseases, she immediately started to practise it with single-minded devotion. One month later it was discovered that the infiltration had been assimilated. Then she became more confident of the effect of *Qigong*. She got up at 5 every morning and persisted in practising it very conscientiously. After three months' practice, her condition improved obviously. She had a better appetite, no longer suffered from insomnia and had never caught cold ever since. When she was reexamined in Nov. 1979, her pulmonary cavity had entiredly disappeared.

Ⅳ. Prescriptions for and Case Studies of Splenic and Gastric Diseases

The spleen governs blood and is responsible for transport and conversion and for the growth of muscles and the activities of extremities. The "spleen and stomach" are called the "essentials for the growth of the human body". The common symptoms of splenic and gastric diseases are : constipation, abdominal distension and pain, tenderness, indigestion, distension of stomach and epigastric upset, regurgiation and vomiting, edema, haemorrhage and foot atrophy. The major *Qigong* pattern used to treat splenic and gastric diseases is the Toe-Raised Transport and Conversion Pattern. The Blowing Method to Strengthen the Kidney and the Blowing Method to Strengthen the Liver, Spleen and Lung should also be added.

For patients with constipation, the Relaxed and Quiescent *Qi*-Regulating Pattern should also be added with the stick turning outward. And for patients with diarrhea, the stick should turn inward.

For patients with insomnia, Head-Massaging and Mind-Tranquilizing Pattern and the Kidney-Massaging and Essence-Benefiting Pattern should be added.

Pose the center of the palm upward for patients with gastroptosis.

Pronounce the Chinese character "gong" for patients with distinctive splenic diseases and pronounce the Chinese character "dong" for patients with distinctive gastric diseases. Pronounce ten times each. First, pronounce three times, and then increase to the sixth time and the tenth time if the patient does not feel uncomfortable.

Massage of the spleen should be done at the spleen region which is below the hypochondrium. And massage of the stomach should be done in the middle of the gastric region.

Case

Patient: Cao, male, 21.

The patient was sick with gastroptosis for more than

7 years and in the last three years his condition got very serious. He was once hospitalized for treatment. In March, 1980, he was diagnosed as gastroptosis (8 cm). His symptoms were insomnia, poor appetite, shortness of breath, emaciation with yellowish complexion, and general weakness. He had to wear a gastral support to hold up his stomach. After he took up Qigong exercise, he persistently got up at 4 a. m. and practised Qigong for four hours every day. In accordance with the sequence of Qigong patterns he emphasized the Toe-Raised Transport and Conversion Pattern. In the evening he practised the Yongquan Point Massage in addition to the Head Massage and the Relaxed and Quiescent Qi-Regulating Pattern. After three months' practice, his condition improved greatly: His appetite was good; his complexion gained colour; he could walk with a free and forceful pace and his gastral support was removed. Later he was reexamined in a hospital, which proved that his condition had improved greatly: The gastroptosis reduced from 8 cm to 3 cm.

V. Prescriptions for and Case Studies of Renal Diseases

The kidney controls the essence of life and stores the original yin and yang. It is most encouraged to reenforce it and any wasteful dissipation should be avoided. Most of the diseases of the kidney belong to asthenia-syndromes. Symptoms of deficiency of kidney-yang are cold in the extremities, listlessness, lassitude in the knees and loins, frequent micturation, impotence; symptoms of deficiency of kidney-yin are involuntary emission and premature ejaculation,

253

drops after urination, frequent micturation or urinary incontinence, hypoacusis, light-headedness, dry mouth and night sweat, edema and so on.

The major *Qigong* patterns used to treat renal diseases are the Blowing Method to Strengthen the Kidney, the Toe-Raised Transport and Conversion Pattern and the Kidney-Massaging and Essence-Benefiting Pattern.

For patients who suffer from deficiency of kidney-energy and who gasp for breath at any motion, the Blowing Method to Strengthen the Lung should be added.

For patients with deficiency of *yin* essence and lassitude of the knees and lions, the Relaxed and Quiescent *Qi*-Regulating Pattern should be added.

For patients with light-headedness, tinnitus or deafness, the Head-Massaging and Mind-Tranquilizing Pattern should be added.

Patients with renal diseases pronounce the Chinese character "yu". First pronounce 3 times and then increase to the sixth time when the patient is adapted to it.

Case

Patient: Wang, female, 56, works in a broadcasting bureau.

The patient began to suffer from hypertension in 1956 and in 1967 she was diagnosed as having frequently-occurring aorto-arteritis and stenosis of renal artery. In 1972, her urinary albumin was positive with + + + and her blood pressure rose up to 230/120. Radioisotope therapy revealed moderate damage of her renal function. In 1976, she was given a renal scan which indicated atrophy of both kidneys while the chart of her cerebral blood stream indicated a functional change. Then the patient suffered from such a severe pain in the head that even large doses of analgesics produced no effect. Her symptoms included insomnia, tinnitus and light-headedness, palpitation and shortness of breath, thoracic pain and tightness in the chest, night micturation 5-6 times, abnormal sweating due to general debility, low fever in the afternoon, ESR 110mm/h. She had an appetite for only two *liang* of food each day. She visited many hospitals and received various kinds of treatment but the effect was not satisfactory.

After practising *Qigong*, her symptoms basically disappeared. She had a much better appetite; she could sleep well; her resistance to diseases was built up. Symptoms such as night frequent micturation, tinnitus, pain in the back and loins all disappeared. In the past, her lower limbs were cold and numb, but now they were warm. Her haemochrome rose from 5 g to 10.5 g, with normal WBC. There was no longer a strong smell of uric acid from her nasal cavity as she had before. The changes are shown in the following table:

item	before practice	after practice
symptoms	severe headache, insomnia; sleep on drugs, night micturation 5-6 times, appetite for 2 *liang* of food daily	no headache, sound sleep without drugs, no night micturation, appetite for 1 *jin* of food daily
haemochrome	5 g	10.5 g

item	before practice	after practice
cholesterol	270mg%	160mg%
urinary albumin	++++	stable at +-++
blood pressure	230/120mmHg	160-170/90mmHg

Ⅵ. Prescriptions for and Case Studies of Miscellaneous Diseases

Miscellaneous diseases are either complicated multiple diseases or diseases the classification of which has not yet been made. As the *Qigong* therapy takes the human body as a whole in treatment, it can cure difficult and complicated diseases from various angles.

For instance, it seems that atrial fibrillation can be included in the category of heart diseases. However, some atrial fibrillations are closely related to the nerves so they may also be included in the category of miscellaneous diseases. The cerebrovascular accidents may be included in the category of cardiovascular diseases, but they are different from the ordinary heart diseases and thus, may also be included in the category of miscellaneous diseases. Miscellaneous diseases are too many to be mentioned here in detail. So only a few cases are exemplified here for the reference of *Qigong* practitioners.

Case No. 1

Patient: Zhang, male, 32, works at a factory of special radio equipment in the town of Hebi, Henan Province.

In 1975, the patient suddenly became staggering in walking and gradually became mentally listless. A relative of the patient said that there had been members of the family who suffered from the same disease for generations. The patient thought he was suffering from an incurable disease and thus lost hope and confidence.

After practising Qigong for some time, the patient came to know the fundamental tenets that diseases are caused by obstruction of the circulation of the vital energy and blood, imbalance of the yin and yang and nervousness. He learned and applied various Qigong patterns to build up his constitution. Gradually he got used to getting up on time and persisted in practising Qigong. Now he has completely recovered mentally. He walks with firm steps and no longer feels tired when working.

Case No. 2

Patient: Gao, male, 43, works at Beijing Food Industry Research Institute.

The patient began to have constant palpitations in 1978. In March, 1979, he was diagnosed as paroxysmal atrial fibrillation, of which severe attack would last more that 4 hours. In October, the same year, sinusoid and atrial premature systole occurred—8-9 attacks a minute for severe occasions. His heart arrest was accompanied by headache, perspiration, general weakness, tightness in the chest, and pain in the left region of the heart with the rhythm of heart over 170 beats a minute.

During the first 3 months of his Qigong practice, he

did all the five fundamental *Qigong* patterns. And then, from the 4th month on, he only practised the Blowing Method to Strengthen the Liver, the Spleen and the Lung which belong to the Breath-Regulating and Qi-Reen-forcing Pattern. Each method was practised for more than 20 minutes, totalling 1.5-2 hours a day. He felt happy and comfortable and had a sensation of *Qi* during the exercise. For an occasional attack of atrial fibrillation, he would practise a set of the Breath-Regulating and Qi-Reenforcing Pattern and the Toe-Raised Transport and Conversion Pattern which would bring his heart rhythm to normal. After 5 months' practice, he was able to work full-time.

Case No. 3

Patient: Yan, male, 55, is a cadre retired from Guanghua Material Factory.

In 1973, while carrying something heavy, the patient got his right foot injured and his lumbar and thoracic vertebra seriously twisted. As affected by the sequela, his condition became weaker and weaker. Early in 1977, he got hypertension. His maximum blood pressure was 210/130 mmHg. He had dizziness, palpitation and abnormal sweat. Sometimes he fainted. In 1979, he was ill with thrombus. He had hemiplegia and eye-twitching and distortion of the mouth. After hospitalization and treatment, his condition improved, but he still had numbness in his right lower limb and could not walk without a stick. So he was retired.

After practising the Toe-Raised Transport and Conversion Pattern, the Breath-Regulating and Qi-Reenforcing Pattern and so on, he was fully recovered from the sequela of the thrombus. Three months later, he was seen walking without the stick.

Ⅶ. **Prescriptions for and Case Studies of Tumours (Cancers)**

For different positions of tumour, different additional *Qigong* patterns should be performed. For example, for patients with tumours the Fast Blowing Method and the Open-Mouth Breathing-Out Method should be performed in addition to the five basic *Qigong* patterns in accordance with their pathological conditions. Here are some additional *Qigong* patterns for different patients: For patients with carcinoma of the lung, add the Method to Strengthen the Lung and the Method to Strengthen the Kidney; for patients with adnocarcinoma, add the Blowing Method to Strengthen the Lung and pronounce the Chinese character "shang"; for patients with cerebral carcinoma, add the Method to Strengthen the Kidney and the Blowing Method to Strengthen the Heart and pronounce the Chinese charater "duo"; for patients with nasopharyngeal carcinoma, add the Blowing Method to Strengthen the Lung and pronounce the Chinese character "shang"; for patients with carcinoma of the large intestine, add the Blowing Mehthod to Strengthen the Lung and pronounce the Chinese character "shang"; for patients with carcinoma of the small intestine, add the Blowing Method to Strengthen the Heart and pronounce the Chinese character "zheng"; for patients with carcinoma of the gallbladder, add the Blowing Method to Strengthen the Lung, the Liver and the Spleen and pronounce the Chinese character "guo"; for patients with carcinoma of the urinary bladder and uterus, add the Blowing Method to Strengthen the Kidney and pronounce the Chinese character "yu"; for patients with dermal carcinoma, add the Blowing Method to Strengthen the Lung, the Liver and the Spleen and pronounce the Chinese character "shang".

So long as one performs the *Qigong* patterns in accordance with the instructions given in the "viscera-state doctrine" of the *Qigong* theory, good results will be achieved and diseases cured.

The following are some cases for reference.

Case No. 1

Patient: Wang, male, 54, works at the General Company of Bus Service.

In the spring of 1980, the patient suddenly lost consciousness and he came to himself only after an emergency treatment in a hospital. By means of cerebral radiography and marrow analysis, the diagnosis was confirmed as tumour of the cerebral artery. His doctor suggested that he be operated on but he refused. By the time he left the hospital, he was very weak. His hands were feeble and quivering and his feces incontinent. He could hardly take care of himself in his daily life. He was in low spirits and his family members were also worried.

On Fed.14, 1981, the patient began to practise *Qigong*, mainly performing the Breath-Regulating and Qi-Reenforcing Pattern and the Toe-Raised Transport and Conversion Pattern. He felt strength in his legs and could walk about alone. Incontinence of feces and urine disappeared. When he went back to the hospital for reexamination, the doctor said that he could not find anything abnormal with him. Now he feels quite well and rarely catches cold. His mental state has also greatly improved. He has resumed work.

Case No. 2

Patient: Wang, female, 33, works at the Hospital of Beijing Steel works.

Here is a case of metastatic carcinoma of cerebral glands. Ten weeks after her practice of *Qigong* therapy, the patient's condition improved greatly. The changes are shown in the following table.

before practice	after practice
1. distention in the head, bulging eyeballs	1. these symptoms apparently subsided, recurrence only on performing the Fast Blowing Method, but easily controlled by *daoyin*
2. serious hyperplasia of mammary glands to the front edge of armpit	2. hyperplasia has basically disappeared
3. general weakness, support needed when going up and down the staircase	3. feeling at ease and strength in the legs
4. poor appetite, 2 *liang* of food a meal	4. great improvement in appetite, often feels hungry and a gain of 4-5 *jin* of body weight
5. dull pain around the navel, often has to lie on stomach at night	5. abdominal pain has disappeared
6. white secretion at eye corners	6. white secretion has disappeared

Case No. 3

Patient: Liu, male, 48, works in the First Sanitation Vehicles Factory of Beijing.

In the past year and more, the patient had difficulty in breathing, expiratory dispnea, coughing and expectorating frequently. X-Ray examination revealed that his upper left lung did not dilate and there was a swelling in the bronchus. He was diagnosed as having pulmonary carcinoma and he was greatly depressed. Through the practice of Qigong in combination with some other treatments, he gained strength and began to breathe effortlessly. The pain in the back subsided and thoracic tightness decreased. Further X-Ray examination showed that his left lung had already dilated and the swelling in the bronchus disappeared. Subsequent reexaminations showed the same results. Now, he has resumed full-time work.

Case No. 4

Patient: Zhang, female, 53, works at the Designing Office of the District Planning Commission of Hami, Xinjiang Autonomous Region.

Patient was sick with carcinoma in the vulva in Jan. 1980. Nine months after an operation, the focus of infection was metastasized to the lung with a 8 cm shadow on it. She had symptoms such as coughing, panting, low blood pressure, spitting blood, fatigue, listlessness and poor appetite. Laboratory tests showed a deficiency of the functions of the heart, kidney and liver and active cancer cells. Her condition was too bad to permit chemotherapy or radiotherapy.

She accepted the self-controlled *Qigong* therapy on Jan. 13, 1981. After one month's practice, she could have 7–8 *liang* of starch food a day. Her coughing disappeared and she no longer spat any blood. She rarely caught cold.

After two months' practice, she took a favourable turn in her mental state. When doing *Qigong* exercise, her arms had a tingling sensation and her hands were warm. She felt as if there were electric currents inside her body, functioning as *daoyin*. So she became more confident of the effect of *Qigong*. She managed to get up at 3–4 o'clock every morn ing and persisted in practising *Qigong* for 4–5 hours each day despite of bad weather. In April, 1981, she went to the hospital for reexamination. X-Ray of her chest showed: the tumour in the lung decreased by 2/3 in size.

Case No. 5

Patient: Zhang, works in the Mineral Bureau of Hebi, Henan Province.

About ten years ago, the patient noticed some red rashes like eczema in his groin, which gave him a lot of trouble. He visited many hospitals and received various kinds of treatment but no improvement was effected. Later, the rashes grew to the size of a walnut. The patient was getting thinner apparently and his body weight decreased to no more than 110 *jin*. Because of the pain, he had difficulty in walking. He was examined in a hospital and diagnosed as having scale-shaped epithelioma. So, he was operated on and one of his lymph nodes in the groin was removed. Examination of the lymph showed that there was a metastasis, and adenocarcinoma was developed. Later the metastasis spread from the exterior to the interior part of the body. The doctors held that a major operation must be performed and suggested that the patient's infected leg be removed. Thinking that he could not live long even with the leg removed, the patient refused the operation. In May, 1981, the patient accepted the Self-Controlled Therapy. He got up early every morning, doing the fast breathing exercisetwo inhalations followed by one exhalation. After two months' practice, he not only felt well, but also found his WBC count stable even after the radiotherapy. He gained 15 *jin* in his body weight. The lymph node, which was as big as a finger tip, was now much smaller and softer. After three months' practice the lymph node reduced to half of the original size and at the end of the tenth month, the lymph node disappeared completely. Now he weighs 157 *jin* in body weight. On the eve of the Spring Festival of 1982 when he was reexamined by renal and hepatic scanning, barium meal radiography of the intestines and stomach, proctoscopy and X-Ray of the lung, everything was found normal.

中国气功疗法

张明武　孙星垣　著

杨恩堂　姚秀清　译

中国山东科学技术出版社出版
（中国济南南郊宾馆西路）
中国山东新华印刷厂潍坊厂印刷
（中国潍坊工农路 99 号）
中国国际图书贸易总公司发行
（中国国际书店）
（北京 399 信箱）
1985 年 第 1 版
编号：（英）14195·194
00650
14—E—1958P